THE BOOK OF
EXECUTIVE
HEALTH

A GUIDE FOR MEN AND WOMEN
EXECUTIVES WHO WANT TO LIVE LONGER

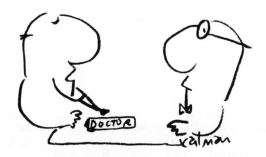

TIMES BOOKS <u>AND</u> THE BRITISH MEDICAL
ASSOCIATION

A SPECTRUM BOOK

PRENTICE-HALL INC. Englewood Cliffs, New Jersey 07632

Library of Congress Cataloging in Publication Data
Main entry under title:

The Book of executive health.

  (A Spectrum Book)
  Includes index.
    1. Health. 2. Executives—Health programs. 3. Job
stress. I. The Times, London. II. British Medical
Association.
RA776.5.B66 1981   613'.088658   80-28584
ISBN 0-13-080010-4
ISBN 0-13-080002-3 (pbk.)

Editorial/production supervision by Louise M. Marcewicz
Cover design by Diane Saxe
Manufacturing buyer: Cathie Lenard

Previously published under the title *The BMA Book of Executive Health.*

The passage on pp. 74-75 is taken from Dr. Charles K. Friedberg's paper in *Circulation* (1972), 46, 1037, by permission of the American Heart Association, Inc.

A SPECTRUM BOOK

10 9 8 7 6 5 4 3 2 1

Printed in the United States of America

PRENTICE-HALL INTERNATIONAL, INC., *London*
PRENTICE-HALL OF AUSTRALIA PTY. LIMITED, *Sydney*
PRENTICE-HALL OF CANADA, LTD., *Toronto*
PRENTICE-HALL OF INDIA PRIVATE LIMITED, *New Delhi*
PRENTICE-HALL OF JAPAN, INC., *Tokyo*
PRENTICE-HALL OF SOUTHEAST ASIA PTE. LTD., *Singapore*
WHITEHALL BOOKS LIMITED, *Wellington, New Zealand*

CONTENTS

2191409

FOREWORD

Certain occupations that involve responsibility and important decision-making, such as that of an executive, carry inherent stresses which constitute particular hazards to health. This book comprehensively and concisely describes the various factors that are potentially stressful, and the various means of coping with stress and with illnesses that may be aggravated by or associated with it.

Stress is, however, a part of normal experience and in moderation can serve a useful purpose by promoting arousal and enhancing effort and alertness, helping a person to maintain high standards of work and behavior. But if it is severe and prolonged, excess stress may tax an individual's capacity to adjust to such an extent that behavioral or bodily changes take place that may lead to the development of disease. The disease may be physical, psychiatric, or psychosomatic.

An important element in the prevention of such diseases may lie in the ability of the individual to be honest with himself about his lifestyle, to be realistic about what he can reasonably expect to achieve. Illness itself is likely to lead to further stress, and perhaps to further illness. An understanding of the likely reasons for illness, its symptoms and treatment, helps to promote an awareness of what can be done to maintain one's own health. This book is essential reading for executives and others in positions of responsibility who would like to minimize the risk of succumbing to the effects of stress. It contains a wealth of practical information regarding the promotion of positive physical and mental health, and wisdom regarding exercise, diet, rest, sleep, and the dangers of excessive drinking and abuse of drugs. Indeed, it is a valuable source of information for everyone, not only in the prevention of ill health and disease but also in encouraging individuals to enjoy positive good health.

W. Linford Rees
CBE, DSc, MD, FRCP, FRCPsych, FACP(Hon), DPM.

CONTRIBUTORS

Margaret Allen
Features Editor and an Assistant Editor of *The Times*; part-time member of the Equal Opportunities Commission

Graham Bennette, MB, BChir
Medical Services Secretary, Royal Society of Medicine

Dr. Beulah Bewley, MSc, MA, MD, MFCM
Senior Research Fellow Department of Social Medicine and Clinical Epidemiology, St. Thomas's Hospital

T. H. Bewley, MD, FRCPI, FRCPsych, DPM
Consultant Physician, St. Thomas's Hospital; member of Medical Council on Alcoholism; member of Institute of Study of Drug Addiction

Ivor Felstein, MB, ChB
Department of Geriatrics, Bolton District General Hospital; member of the British Geriatric Society and Geriatric Care Association

John Hampton, DPhil, DM, FRCP
Reader in Medicine and Consultant Physician, University of Nottingham Medical School; member of the Atherosclerosis Discussion Group and British Cardiac Society

Clifford Hawkins, MD, FRCP
Consultant Physician of United Birmingham and mid-Worcestershire Hospital; Lecturer in Clinical Medicine, University of Birmingham

W. T. Jones, MD, FFCM, DIH, DPH, MFOM
First Director General of the Health Education Council. At present District Community Physician, Brent Health District; Principal Medical Adviser, Whitbread Limited

P. G. F. Nixon, FRCP
Consultant Cardiologist, Charing Cross Hospital; member of the British Cardiac Society

I. Michael Ormerod, MB, BChir
Medical Officer, Commercial Union Insurance Company Limited

John Pollitt, MD, FRCP, FRCPsych, DPM
Physician-in-Charge, Department of Psychological Medicine, St. Thomas's Hospital; awarded Gaskell Gold Medal of the Royal Medico-Psychological Association

A. J. Smith, BM, BCh
Deputy Editor of the *British Medical Journal*; Medical Correspondent of *The Times*

Eric J. Trimmer, MB, BS, MRCGP
General practitioner; Editor of *British Journal of Sexual Medicine*; Medical Editor of *Medical News*

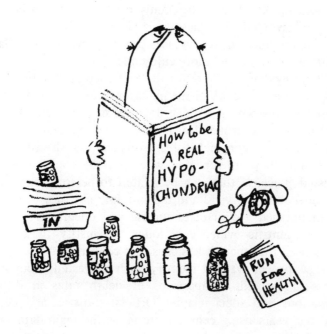

chapter 1

EXECUTIVES: THE REAL HEALTH RISKS

No one suggests that the work of an executive carries hazards of the same magnitude as that of a coal-miner or of a deep-sea diver. Even so, there are some risks inherent in an executive's way of life that need to be understood. Serious illness causing sudden death, early disability or premature retirement, is not a random stroke of fate; the predisposing factors can be recognized and avoided. The message is clear: help yourself. Health can be maintained, many diseases can be prevented or delayed, and life made fuller and more enjoyable.

What evidence is there for the existence of specific occupational hazards in the job of the manager or executive? Most of it is based on hearsay. A sudden death after a particularly tough board meeting, a stroke after a demanding overseas sales trip, a suicide when a contract folds—everyone has heard of such events, and they are repeated whenever the topic of health is discussed. Because they can be related to personal experiences these anecdotes are vivid and meaningful, and they have gradually encouraged a climate of unease and uncertainty. In fact, if solid scientific evidence is sought to justify these fears it may be seen that there is less cause for concern.

The proper way to identify such suggested occupational threats is through comparisons of death rates in different occupations and social classes. Official statistics are prepared every ten years using census material as the main data source. Managerial-executive jobs are difficult to categorize in the precise way used for clergymen, doctors, or lawyers, as the job is so variable. The broad message is nevertheless optimistic. Generally, the death rate for executives is as good as, for example, that of lawyers, and much better than that of skilled workers, who in turn are more favored than unskilled workers. On the other hand executives' mortality is not as good as that of clergymen or higher civil servants. Deaths of executives from diabetes, suicide, and diseases associated with high blood pressure are more common than among others in the same social class—though they are still less frequent than among manual workers. All in all, the figures give little help one way or the other to the individual who is seeking guidance, except to make clear that in terms of survival it is preferable to be better educated and better paid.

Not surprisingly, executives wanting more specific guidance on their health have looked for expert advice, and in the last two decades there has been a spectacular growth in screening examinations of various types, regular checkups, counseling sessions, physical exercise routines, weight watching, smoking control clinics, and so on. Without a doubt, all these measures can benefit individuals—and for most people that is a good enough test of their validity. The medical rationale behind them is explained directly and indirectly in the chapters that follow.

Nevertheless, there is still a lot of medical skepticism about the value of these procedures. For the scientist, any threat to health should be measurable in terms of increased deaths, illness, absence from work, hospital admissions, and doctors' attendances. These stringent tests cannot, however, come to terms with the complex of cultural, behavioral, and social factors which make up the quality of life.

Probably the tools that have been used to explore these influences on health have been too imprecise and inappropriate for the job in hand. If, as seems likely, the hazards to the executive are not in the physical environment—dust, noise, pollution—but in the behavioral-cultural milieu involving personal behavior, then different tests may be needed. Conventional methods of medical exploration may not be capable of revealing these less obvious threats. Medicine has to proceed pragmatically, without undue haste, yet with the protection of the individual in a changing world in mind. Equally, the potential patient who is out to protect himself must accept that he can act only on the evidence available.

One of the aims of this book is, then, to give an account of contemporary medical attitudes and the conclusions which follow from them, so that the reader can take appropriate steps. At this moment dogma has little place on a map of uncertainty, but there are enough firm and prominent features on it for any comprehending traveler.

RESPONSIBILITY AND STRESS

In any industrial organization the executives are valuable capital assets because of their long training, their acquired skills, and their expensively obtained experience. It is sometimes thought that the higher an executive progresses up the managerial tree, the greater is the stress, and the more vulnerable he becomes to illness. In fact the opposite may be the case: the successful executive may be less heavily stressed than the man passed over for promotion. The hazards of the executive life are unlike the more conventional occupational risks to health—they must be presumed to be social and behavioral, rather than chemical or physical, in origin. Conventional investigatory methods are of little value in their study. There are many immeasurables present, and the behavioral sciences have yet to develop any readily applicable measures of social relationships which compare with the methods of measurement used in classical occupational medicine. The experimental techniques of sociology, psychology, and social anthropology are as yet relatively crude, and as sciences they still await their Newton.

The executive is required to exercise his skills in the solution of specific problems, and these skills are the product of formal education, experience, and innate aptitudes, combined to produce qualities such as wisdom and foresight. Using these skills (consciously or unconsciously) the competent executive reduces problems to a limited number of abstract concepts, and this being done, uses the process of analogy to deduce alternative solutions for immediate problems. These solutions are weighed one against the other, and one is eventually selected as being the most appropriate to the circumstances. From this point on, the executive is concerned with justifying the solution to other people and ensuring that it is carried out, usually by subordinates. It is during this process of formulating and applying the solution to the problem that stresses of various types arise.

Some degree of stress seems to be necessary to add zest to an existence which might otherwise be only humdrum. We have no way of measuring the amount of stress which is ideal for the continued health of businesspeople. More needs to be known about their habits, motivations, actions, and responses to stimuli, and above all about the effects that different levels and manners of authority have upon these different types of personality.

Conflict is produced when two or more apparently incompatible tensions compete with one another, and where decisions have to be made, there is always potential conflict. Most commonly this results when a choice has to be made between a theoretical, ideal, but unattainable solution and a practical, political, workaday solution which may be less worthy of the individual's personal ideals. Nowadays there may be more interests than ever to consider. The democratic climate of contemporary industrial management produces a host of social, political, and economic considerations and human relationships that have to be weighed in decision-making. Conflict can, therefore, hardly ever be avoided, and ethical and moral dilemmas are only too frequent.

Frustration is a second psychological feature constantly appearing throughout executive life. Having made a decision by reconciling conflicts, the executive has to persuade others to accept the decision and to act upon it. Frustration follows when others cannot or will not accept this solution or when having apparently accepted it they fail, for various reasons, to take the action necessary to make the decision effective.

Many situations brought to the executive for solution

appear at first sight to be insoluble. This appearance of insolubility may produce both conflict and frustration. From these emotions spring subsidiary responses of anxiety, fear, and guilt.

In addition to the stresses inherent in decision-making, there may be subsidiary social burdens which can directly and indirectly influence physical fitness—and as a result impair the mental qualities needed for full and effective command. Among the most familiar are irregular time schedules, the effects of travel, and insufficient and indigestible meals often interspersed with hurried snacks and accompanied by quantities of alcohol and nicotine. Dyspepsia, insomnia, and irritability follow, and are often the first signs of unhealthiness. Indeed, when all these precipitating and predisposing factors are considered, complete breakdown may seem remarkably uncommon.

To remain healthy, then, the executive needs the resilience to shoulder insoluble problems, the stamina to carry them still unsolved for long periods, an unimpaired equanimity which allows him or her to look at their insolubility fearlessly, objectively, and with calm, and to digest them and produce alternative solutions for them.

There are, however, varying degrees of resistance to the burdens of office; some form of biological self-selection may operate which allows only innately healthier people to reach the higher and lonelier eminences of responsibility. It may be that only those with built-in resistance to stress succeed most dramatically in modern business life. If this is so, it seems logical to concentrate medical preventive procedures upon the second level of executives and on those younger persons with apparent ability. Those who have got to the top are there because of their special toughness, and they have already passed the selection tests of time and experience. Those who are in the middle reaches of this modern variant on the survival of the fittest may be most in need of medical attention.

SYMPTOMS OF STRESS

The unhealthy executive does not have, or has at least temporarily lost, a resistance to stress. Loss of self-assurance is often the first sign of unhealthiness, and may be shown by failure to reach clear and effective decisions. At the same time the unhealthy executive may show loss of confidence in subordinates, and will ask for more and more information before reaching a decision—and there may even be a tendency to question the validity of this information. All this adds up to procrastination. Such indecision and hesitancy may well superficially appear as over-activity and can sometimes be mistaken for 'drive' until it becomes clear that less, rather than more, effective action is resulting.

An over-stressed executive may try to concentrate more and more power closely within his own hands; only minutiae are devolved upon subordinates, and as a result the structure of the whole organization begins to disintegrate. Subordinates feel slighted, and frustration affects the whole hierarchy with discontent.

The harassed executive is now in a vicious cycle. Responsibility cannot be devolved, no one is trusted, and more work, requiring more decisions, is fed to him. Work has become so pressing that holidays are refused, and the psychological disturbance may have penetrated sufficiently deeply for physical symptoms to develop.

Means of Escape

This state of mind often shows itself as repeated short sick-leaves—and illness can indeed offer an avenue of temporary escape. The wounds have been suffered in the course of the job and can be sufficient to allow for a period of rest. Beyond this point, the cooperation of colleagues may begin to fail, and the sick executive becomes self-pitying; over-activity is replaced by apathy and depression. Verbal output increases, as does alcohol intake; technical jargon and glib catch-phrases replace considered and original thoughts and judgments. Intellect remains unimpaired but its application fails, and memory plays tricks.

At the end of the process the loss of skills and abilities affects self-esteem. This has largely been built upon pride in skills and aptitudes, and when they demonstrably fail the personality as a whole may begin to disintegrate. Intervention is urgent at this stage if health is to be restored—and if lasting damage is not to occur in both social and business contexts.

EARLY DETECTION PAYS DIVIDENDS

The logic behind the concept of periodic health examinations as a health maintenance procedure seems impeccable, yet many doctors have doubts about their value. As yet there is little convincing evidence that they are effective in detecting unsuspected disease at a stage when it is still reversible. However, the concept appeals strongly to many medical and lay minds, and has enthusiastic support.

Unfortunately the topic is muddled with problems of definition—when, for example, is an abnormality sufficiently severe or established to be called a disease? The existence and discovery of large numbers of variations from 'normal' proves nothing. Any regular examination of an aging biological organism, if thoroughly and carefully performed, must reveal the process of decline and decay. The aim of periodic examinations should be essentially curative—the early detection of disease and its subsequent treatment—in the hope that the course of the illness can be favorably influenced. When strict scientific criteria are applied to the results of screening programs, however, the results have been disappointing.

The same doubts do not apply to specific tests for diseases known to be related to a particular industry. The specific routine examination has a proved and time-honored place in preventive medicine. Whenever occupational hazards have been shown to produce specific clinical and laboratory changes the extent of the environmental risk can be estimated and controlled. But the periodic medical examination is most often applied in situations where a hazard is only dimly suspected, and where the responses it may produce are distributed over the whole wide field of clinical medicine. There is here no definite and proven relationship between environment and response. The indices are nonspecific and their significance vague.

More knowledge is needed about the early clinical forms of diseases, and particularly about the earliest biochemical changes which may be detectable by routine screening procedures. It is perhaps in this latter field that the greatest hope lies for the early detection of disease.

LOOKING AFTER YOURSELF

While we wait for these advances in knowledge, however, there is still a mass of medical advice that can be given in the form of education to those at risk. Prevention holds out far better prospects than does any hope of early detection of symptomless disease. There is now abundant evidence to show that individuals can do most good by concentrating on their own health maintenance. The ultimate aim is not simply a longer life but a fuller and healthier one, free of illness and its attendant disabilities. The dominant causes of illness and death can be influenced by our own behavior in controlling what we eat and drink, in the use of tobacco, alcohol and other drugs, and in a sensible balance between work, leisure, and physical and mental activity.

Our attitude toward our own state of health is sometimes surprisingly passive; the intention of this book is to demonstrate how much can be done to maintain good health by the application of common sense and a rational approach.

chapter 2

EVERYDAY HEALTH PROBLEMS

When we are in good health we tend not to notice it. We take for granted a normal feeling of well-being, energy, alertness, and a general interest in life. Sleep is no problem, and although it may be more difficult to get up on some mornings than on others, the first restorative cup of coffee or tea puts us straight back on track. Illness or disease, however, makes an immediate impact on our normal working day. How can the common symptoms of day-to-day illness most easily be controlled?

COUGHS, COLDS, AND COMPLICATIONS

Symptoms of the common cold vary enormously. Sometimes the nose is the most severely affected region, when a streaming cold makes life a misery as well as being antisocial. Instead of having to blow the nose to clear it just once or twice a day, a packet of tissues becomes an absolute necessity. Some colds affect the throat, which feels dry and rough, and makes swallowing painful. Others go down into the chest, frequently affecting first the larynx, when there is difficulty in speaking, especially in producing a normal-sounding voice. Further down still the inflammation may reach the trachea, causing soreness in the center of the chest and pain with deep breathing.

Perhaps rather more commonly than colds getting down to the chest, the infection may spread up into the sinuses, leading to sinusitis. The sinuses are air spaces continuous with the lining of the nose and throat. They hollow out several of the bones of the skull, notably the frontal bones and the maxillary bones (the bones of the cheeks), primarily to reduce the weight of the head—if these bones in the face and the head were solid, the head would be very difficult to support on the shoulders. The sinuses have another function: They increase and to some extent produce the timbre of the voice. When there is no resonance in the sinuses the voice sounds nasal and tinny.

Colds really pose two problems: first, whether to go to work or to stay at home, and second, what to do about the symptoms. Colds are of course very infectious, but in all probability the peak period of infectiousness occurs before the onset of obvious symptoms. All the evidence suggests that staying at home to protect colleagues at work is pointless. Two people can be practically tied together in experimental conditions in an attempt to give one the other's cold, without any success; the medical view nowadays is that coughs and sneezes may spread some diseases but not the common cold. Doctors have even tried introducing the nasal secretions of somebody who has a cold into the nose of somebody who has not, but once again the infection does not spread. You do not catch colds that way.

The decision about whether or not to go to work really depends on how the individual feels. If the cold is accompanied by a rise in the patient's temperature, by aches and pains in the limbs, or if it becomes difficult to concentrate, it is probably best to stay at home. Furthermore, someone with a cold at this stage should avoid getting chilled; in some way chilling lowers the general resistance of the body, so a simple cold in the nose may become complicated by bronchitis or pneumonia.

Treating a Cold

Treatments for colds are legion. Most doctors take nothing for a cold (unless it is a little whisky or rum, if they are so inclined). A dose of aspirin or aspirin-free substitute often makes a cold feel a little more comfortable, particularly if there is a headache or other aching. Yet almost every television commercial break shows some magic cure for colds, in which people have a sip of something when they go to bed at night and moments later are shown with their colds having disappeared. In fact there is a handful of medical remedies—some of which can be bought over the druggist's counter—that shrink down the inflamed and soggy mucus membranes which are so troublesome in cases of acute infection. Most of these are best taken at bedtime because they have a sedative effect, and are therefore not helpful to someone struggling to keep going during the day. Whether or not they really make colds go away more quickly, or just promote a rather more comfortable night's sleep, is a matter of debate.

Many people believe that large doses of vitamin C have a dramatic effect on colds; despite twenty years of medical research trials there is still no conclusive evidence that this treatment is any better or worse than the traditional toddies, lemon drinks, or aspirin mixtures. One warning, however: do not mix alcohol and aspirin. The combination may sometimes lead to internal bleeding from inflammation of the stomach lining. If a whisky toddy is felt to be desirable, an aspirin-free substitute should be used rather than aspirin.

Sinus Trouble

Colds that go up into the sinuses may be a real nuisance, since they tend to persist. The sinuses are curiously designed: the little orifice through which the secretions should drain is positioned high up in the walls—a legacy of the days when we walked on all fours. This being the case, there is a clear advantage in taking one of the decongestant types of cold cures at night; the chances are that the sinuses will discharge rather better while the patient is lying down than during the day. Another useful treatment for congested sinuses is inhalation of hot steam containing menthol and eucalyptus.

Nasal drops and inhalers are of more questionable value. They often seem to be habit-forming; and nearly always some sort of rebound reaction occurs—in other words, they shrink the lining of the nose, producing a conspicuous improvement for half an hour or so, but then the stuffiness creeps back again, sometimes feeling worse than before.

Laryngitis

A cough accompanying a cold indicates that the body is putting one of its automatic reflex systems into action and preventing infected mucus from going down the respiratory tract. If the infecting germs get into the larynx, or voice box, the vocal cords become swollen and their efficiency is impaired. First the vocal high notes are lost, and eventually all the voice goes because the cords do not vibrate in the normal way. An attack of laryngitis is likely to limit speech to a whisper.

For anyone with laryngitis, steam inhalations certainly help: large quantities of saturated warm air pass over the larynx, which helps shift the mucus easily. An important rule with laryngitis is not to talk, so it is generally a good idea to take a few days off from work. It is preferable for the sufferer to stay at home and keep quiet—which means not being telephoned by colleagues, to whom the reason for the absence should be explained.

CHEST TROUBLE: TRACHEITIS

Tracheitis, that sore center of the chest, should always be treated with a degree of respect. It means that an infection has passed the natural barrier of the larynx and has got into the chest. The inflammation of the air passages causes secretion of mucus, which has to be coughed up; sometimes a cough mixture will help. One of the expectorant (mucus-producing) cough mixtures is best, as these medicines stimulate the glands lining the trachea to produce thinner, less sticky mucus. The second type of cough mixture—cough linctus—acts by depressing the cough reflex to a certain extent. Linctuses are useful if the cough reflex is causing a dry, painful cough when there is little if any mucus to be coughed up. It is a good idea to reduce this natural reflex a little at night, as coughing is likely to prevent sleep. Expectorant or stimulating cough mixtures are usually taken in very much larger doses than linctuses. They often work very well if taken in hot water, as this helps to shift sticky mucus from the larynx and the trachea by reflex action. Cough medicines really play no part in the treatment of uncomplicated colds. If a cold deteriorates into bronchitis, the doctor's advice should be sought; he may think an antibiotic is needed.

ACHES, PAINS, AND RHEUMATISM

Everybody gets a touch of rheumatism sometimes; the most common type is non-articular or muscular rheumatism. The symptoms do not affect the joints themselves but rather the tissues around joints—ligaments, fibrous tissue, and muscles. The trouble is usually self-inflicted, though it may sometimes be simply accidental or unlucky. It is generally caused by sudden overuse of parts of the body that have not been used for some time: a strenuous game of tennis when one is out of practice; the first bout of energetic gardening in spring. A sensible attitude to the stiffness resulting from this overexertion is to take things easy for a few days and then to try again, being less ambitious and limiting the activity to a reasonable level.

The second time excessive demands are made on the body there is a greater likelihood of, for example, a ligament being torn, which can lead to a whole range of unpleasantly painful conditions from tennis elbow and golfer's wrist to fibrositis, lumbago, or a severely torn muscle. A persistent assumption that it is possible to maintain the same standards as those attained in former years may lead to real trouble.

Despite the minor nature of the injury, it may be completely incapacitating. A torn ligament may well cause such severe pain that there is no alternative to resting in bed. Quite often the symptoms will be severe enough for a doctor to be called in, although there is little he can do beyond advising rest and prescribing painkilling drugs. Applying heat to the affected part—a hot-water bottle, a small electric blanket, a heating pad, or an infra-red lamp—will sometimes help, as may hot baths or showers. But the cornerstone of the treatment is always rest: two, three, or four weeks may be needed before the unpleasant symptoms of nonarticular rheumatism disappear.

DISC TROUBLE

During some activities—digging in the garden is one example—a sudden agonizing pain may be felt in the back and extending down the legs. These symptoms probably mean trouble with a disc—the pad of cartilage between the bones of the spinal column. A slight stretching or distortion of one of the discs causes pain from pressure on one or more spinal nerves, which is why the pain radiates down the legs. These intervertebral discs are responsible for much disability in men and women of all ages. If disc trouble is apparent, it is always necessary to see the doctor, and usually an orthopedic surgeon as well. Sometimes immobilization is required; special exercises may be prescribed; in some cases extension (stretching) of the body is indicated. Painkillers and time off from work are also generally necessary.

A prolapsed intervertebral disc ("slipped disc") can occur if an awkward movement is made when the body is already in an awkward position, but they are frequently to some extent self-inflicted injuries: the usual way for a disc to be damaged is during the lifting of a heavy weight. Such an injury is probably not necessary, since there are safe ways to lift heavy objects which can be easily learned, keeping the back straight and confining the movement to the legs. Straining the back by lifting very heavy objects, pushing up jammed windows, and so forth, should be avoided as attacks of a prolapsed disc are disabling and very uncomfortable.

ARTHRITIS

Arthritis is a quite different problem. Here the damage is in the joints themselves. The three common types are: osteoarthritis, rheumatoid arthritis, and gout. These forms of arthritis are not the sort of disability that can be safely handled at home; all need specialist assessment at regular intervals. Osteoarthritis is to some extent a wear-and-tear disease and is made worse, if not produced, by states of the body that put excessive strain on joints. It used to be found frequently in people who did very heavy work, such as porters and coal-heavers. Obesity, which constantly puts strains on joints that were never designed to withstand them, nowadays seems to be the cause of many cases of osteoarthritis. Many people carry around 20 to 30 pounds of excess weight every day—a load that would make us gasp if it were put in a suitcase.

Rheumatoid arthritis is in many ways an entirely different disease. It is still something of a mystery from the medical point of view, but the consensus is that it is one of the auto-immune diseases. For some reason not yet understood, the body's immune system, which normally protects us against infection and invasion by foreign bodies, suddenly regards certain tissues of our own as foreign to it, and attacks them. When these tissues are the lubricating membranes that line our joints the result is rheumatoid arthritis.

The disease often starts in an insidious way. In the early stages patients feel generally unwell for several weeks. They may have fleeting pains in joints and limbs, tingling in the fingers and arms and sometimes, especially in the case of women, they may become anemic. At some time after these symptoms develop, the arthritic lesions make themselves felt. They usually occur first in the small joints and are therefore most likely to be seen in the fingers and toes. Later, larger joints also become affected.

Gout, the third common type of arthritis, is due to an internal chemical disorder that leads to crystals of uric acid being formed in the tissues. Without treatment the joints and surrounding structures become inflamed and gout deposits occur through the body.

All forms of arthritis are usually best dealt with by a team of doctors in a specialist rheumatism clinic, where the services of a medical rheumatologist, an expert in orthopedic surgery, skilled physiotherapists and occupational therapists, and even remedial gymnasts are available. Each patient has to be thoroughly investigated; this often takes several weeks or even months, as blood counts and various x-ray evaluations are carried out before the team decides the best way of handling the case in order to keep the amount of disability to a minimum.

Unfortunately, rheumatism does make big differences to people's lives; just how big those alterations are depends to some extent on how energetic and well conducted the medical treatment is. Osteoarthritis is being treated more and more by surgical methods, either by the removal of damaged parts of joints, or by the complete replacement of arthritic joints when the disease has become very advanced.

Rheumatoid arthritis is more likely to be treated by a combination of anti-rheumatic drugs, of which there is an increasing number and variety. One of the best drugs for treating rheumatism remains aspirin in one of its many forms. It is a mistake to think that a rheumatologist who recommends aspirin is offering inferior treatment. Aspirin is anti-inflammatory as well as being anti-rheumatic, and it is a painkiller too. No other single drug is so effective. Gout (and other rarer types of arthritis) can nowadays also be controlled by specific drugs which restore the internal chemistry to normal, getting at the root of the trouble. Unfortunately most of these drug treatments require continuous medication if symptoms are not to recur.

EYE TROUBLE

Taking proper care of the eyes is essential to the maintenance of normal good health. Everyone should visit the optician regularly for a checkup on the general condition of the eyes and advice on whether or not glasses are needed. Most middle-aged people become progressively more far-sighted, and there is really no point in their putting off getting glasses merely for the sake of appearance.

Glaucoma
Another advantage of seeing an optician regularly is for a check on the health of less obvious parts of the eye, and in particular the retina at the back of the eyeball. Some of these checks are very important. Perhaps the most serious disease that may go undetected without a regular checkup is glaucoma, a rise in the internal pressure in the eye. For example, in England glaucoma causes some 1500 people to become blind every year, and many more find their vision permanently impaired. The numbers are even worse in the United States. The sad thing about glaucoma is that in well over half the cases diagnosis is made too late for control to be possible. This is because many people, particularly when they are in late middle age, expect their eyes to be substandard and tend to do very little about deterioration in vision.

There are two main types of glaucoma. It is unlikely that anybody would fail to seek medical advice for the rarer form—the acute glaucoma—as the symptoms are startling enough to get anybody to a doctor quickly. There is an agonizing pain in the eye or face together with a sudden loss of vision, often the patient feels very ill and frequently vomits. Unless treatment is prompt and effective, this type of glaucoma can produce a rapid and permanent loss of vision. Many people do, however, have a warning before such a catastrophe. It may take the form of a transient dimness of vision, a halo may be seen around bright lights, there may be recurrent watering or redness of one eye (this, of course, often occurs for much less serious reasons). Women over the age of forty are particularly prone to develop acute glaucoma, and attacks sometimes seem to be precipitated by worry or domestic problems.

The more common type of glaucoma—chronic glaucoma— is more insidious in its approach. Sometimes the warnings are similar to those of the acute variety, but more often the field of vision gradually becomes defective. Most people notice blindness on the nasal side of their vision quite quickly; similarly, a visual defect in the lower half of the field may become apparent- articles at floor level tend to be missed, and the victim stumbles over things he just does not see. Blindness in the upper and outer fields of vision may be ignored, probably because this outside area of vision is less important to us. It can, however, be dangerous, particularly for anyone who drives a car, as he or she may not see an approaching vehicle.

The optician can often diagnose impending glaucoma just by looking into the eyes and by doing special visual field tests. If he suspects something, he will recommend consulting an ophthalmic specialist. With treatment, glaucoma can usually be controlled—and this means preventing blindness.

Cataract

The other major visual problem that tends to get neglected, even now, is cataract—a progressive clouding of the lens at the front of the eye. There still seems to be a sort of folklore among people that cataract is something natural. A quite recent survey reported that a high proportion of patients registered as blind had never received any treatment for their cataract at all.

Cataract shows itself as a gradually diminishing acuteness of vision in the eye, and is unlikely to develop until about the age of fifty. There is no treatment that dissolves a cataract—drops or electrical treatments sometimes still advised by quacks are completely useless.

In the past there was a tendency to leave cataracts until they were sufficiently "advanced" before any attempt was made to remove them. Nowadays advanced techniques of cataract removal and highly sophisticated modifications of the older type of cataract surgery have outdated this attitude, and the advantage of earlier treatment has been accepted.

EAR TROUBLE

The other major sense organ requiring care for the maintenance of average good health is, of course, the ear. There are two main types of deafness—conductive deafness and perceptive deafness. Conductive deafness means that the sound just does not get conducted through the ear drum on to the actual organ of hearing in the way that it should. Often there are the simplest possible causes for this sort of deafness—such as wax in the ears. If someone suddenly starts complaining that he wants the television louder or the radio volume turned up, or just fails to catch what is said to him, he should see a doctor; it should not be accepted as an inevitable part of aging. Wax in the ears can be removed very easily. The doctor may prescribe ear drops in the first instance, which will soften up the wax and make its subsequent removal easier.

There are many other forms of deafness in which early diagnosis is equally important; once again treatment can make a tremendous improvement to the hearing. One of these is otosclerosis—for practical purposes a sort of mini-arthritis affecting the sound-conducting bones within the ear. It results in a progressive loss of hearing, and it is the sort of loss that often makes people feel isolated from their environment. It can affect young as well as middle-aged and more elderly people, but it can be greatly improved by an operation. Finally a word about hearing aids. Hearing aids come in a variety of forms these days: some very tiny miniaturized aids that can be hidden away in a pair of spectacles, others a relatively small behind-the-ear instrument. The advice of an ear, nose and throat (ENT) specialist should always be sought; hearing aids can be bought directly through various commerical channels and shops specializing in the sale of hearing aids, but some of these organizations are more interested in the sale of the aid than in finding the best type of prescription for somebody's deafness.

PREVENTION—A POSITIVE APPROACH

Do health clinics have any positive advantages in maintaining good health? This is perhaps one instance in which women fare better than men. If a woman is registered with her general practitioner for contraceptive purposes, she will automatically receive health checks from time to time. Part of the proper prescription of contraceptives for women is a record of their weight, blood pressure, menstrual history, the state of their pelvic organs, smear tests, and other factors in their general health.

Many companies run special health clinics and schemes for their employees, men as well as women. However, these often involve subjecting people to a battery of rather non-specific physical examinations and laboratory tests which are then given detailed analysis. The aim is to spot disease in a preclinical form before the patient himself knows he is ill, and may be useful in certain circumstances and to monitor blood pressure, weight, and so on. Sometimes quite minor disabilities can also be diagnosed at an early stage before they start adversely to affect good health. Varicose veins provide a good example: Untreated varicose veins are still the cause of a great deal of disability in older people, though treatment can generally cure them. However, the enthusiastic claims sometimes made for the value of an annual checkup should be viewed with some skepticism. There are only a few diseases that can be detected and treated before symptoms have developed, and people who take reasonable care of their health have little need of batteries of sophisticated tests.

Health Farms

The idea of spending a week or two in an establishment which commits visitors to an intensive scheme to improve fitness fast is an attractive one in many ways. There are, however, good and bad health farms, and it is often difficult to distinguish between them merely by comparing glossy brochures. When in doubt it is almost always wise to think that bigger is better and longest established better than the latest one to open its doors.

By and large, the principles behind the treatment are the same. The focus of attention is almost always on losing weight and increasing exercise tolerance. Usually this means a low-calorie diet, no alcohol, no smoking, and a planned regimen of graduated exercise. This, of course, promotes health, especially in the cardiovascular context.

It is possible to attain equally effective results in terms of health in various other ways, but the discipline imposed at a health farm is often more readily acceptable—particularly after the fees have been paid—and it is easier to accept the need to do things we would not normally do or to go without things that would generally prove irresistible.

Health farms gain through the psychological boost of the group and the principle of "What he can do (and put up with) I can do too." They often succeed in making exercise fun and improvement in health a measurable achievement to be proud of; there is no doubt that many people leave health farms much fitter than when they arrived. They may also have lost some excess weight and gained the necessary incentive to lose more, or at least not to put back on what they have lost.

The Value of Exercise

Approached sensibly, the achievements of a visit to a health farm may be followed with equal success in normal life and can make a conspicuous difference to the maintenance of good health and a feeling of well-being. The value of a low carbohydrate (starch and sugar) diet is that the body stores less fat when the starch and sugar intake is low. Exercise is a valuable accompaniment to a weight-reducing diet and should support any attempt to lose weight. The value lies not in increasing energy requirements (the number of calories lost through exercise is generally quite small) but in improving the tone of limb, trunk, and abdominal muscles. There is also some evidence that regular exercise retards the aging process in the arteries of limbs and of the heart. Even a busy executive should try to set aside an appropriate time each day for exercise, which may be either organized or informal.

By "thinking mobile" it is possible to increase the amount of exercise taken each day quite substantially, by using stairs instead of the elevator, for example, by walking instead of driving short distances, and so on. More specific exercise should be taken regularly, rather than in occasional bursts; nor should it be too vigorous, as this may produce fatigue or muscle strain.

Health Foods

Finally a word about health foods. Is there really such a thing—and are the items on sale in special health food shops medically valuable? These shops may be of practical value. A later chapter explains the usefulness of cereal bran, for example, which can help to prevent many unpleasant digestive ailments, particularly later in life; bran is not generally available in supermarkets. Health food shops are often the one place where it is possible to buy fruit juices without added sugar; they sell whole-meal flour that has been ground to keep the maximum bran content; they may have different interesting types of beverages and teas, and decaffeinated coffee. Health food shops often stock more unusual foods which, even if they do not directly improve health, may encourage a healthier and more sensible attitude toward nutritional values and toward the establishment of a properly balanced diet.

COMMON SENSE ABOUT HEALTH

Nobody should expect to feel completely well—energetic, alert, lively—all the time; it is important to apply common sense to maintaining oneself in good health. There will be times when tiredness is unavoidable, but it should be compensated for when time allows by a period of relaxation. Ill health of even a minor kind is inconvenient and often uncomfortable, but has to be accepted as a fact of life. Those who rise on the executive ladder may increasingly come to equate quality with cost, but as far as health is concerned expensive treatment may not necessarily be the right answer. Before approaching specialists it is wise to discuss any problems with one's own general practitioner and get advice on what should be done. The general practitioner has a patient's full records, and will probably know the patient in the context of personal, family, social, and occupational background.

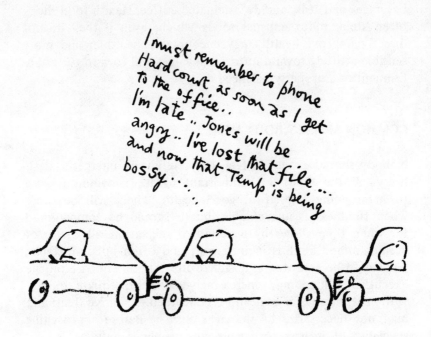

chapter 3
STRESS
AND MENTAL HEALTH

Everyone talks about stress and most people encounter it, but it is still difficult to define. At first glance stress is anything we find problematical, yet most people spend their time solving problems and enjoy doing so.

Apart from the major basic physiological deprivations such as starvation or prolonged sleep loss, there is no set of circumstances that invariably imposes stress on everyone. One man's difficulties are the next man's challenge. One woman delights in opportunities for public speaking which would worry another for weeks. Situations which cause anxiety at the age of nineteen are welcomed at fifty. For many people short periods of stress are enjoyable, as the makers of horror films and the designers of roller coasters and chambers of horror know very well.

Perhaps the crucial feature of undesirable stress is an individual's inability to adjust to an imposed situation. The act of striving to overcome difficulties is usually pleasant and healthy. Achieving the goal is satisfying. Even a temporary loss of the ability to deal with a challenge can lead to further enjoyable efforts to overcome it by getting advice and making more relationships in the process. It is only when it becomes clear that the chances of a change in the situation in reasonable time are remote, and that an individual has lost the capacity to alter it, face it, accept it or deal with it, that stress is likely to prove dangerous.

Stress is no new development, and the reader fortunate enough to be relatively untouched may well ask why greater attention need be paid to it now. The reasons are that the twentieth century has seen enormous changes in the lifestyle and life organization in much of the inhabited world, and the long-term effects of many of these changes are still unknown.

Among the changes which many regard as responsible for much current ill health are the increased speed of movement, communication, and decision, the increased accountability and responsibility of the average citizen, the population explosion with its increasing problems of social relationships and competition, and the growth of new media. Other changes affecting many societies are the effects of increasing state control over what were once personal options, and the concurrent (and probably linked) decline of interpersonal relationships.

Of special importance to executives is the development of the technological age and its reliance on computers, with their purely intellectual approach, unchallengeable, and powerful, yet without human sensitivity.

DEFENSES AGAINST STRESS

Before considering in detail the problems of the executive, it may be helpful to outline the defenses used against stress. Understanding these defenses—based on psychological, anthropological, and, occasionally, mechanical and psychiatric concepts—is invaluable in helping individuals to adjust reasonably happily to the complex stress of modern society. Briefly, capacity to deal with stress depends on:

1. Previous training and skill in handling problems successfully.
2. Morale, in that this determines the strength of endeavor and the likelihood of a satisfactory and satisfying outcome.
3. Psychological defenses. These common mental mechanisms are combined in unique proportions for each individual, forming part of the personality. Although not under voluntary control, use of these mechanisms can be influenced when they would not otherwise operate spontaneously.

   For example, many people have a strong capacity to forget the unpleasant aspects of life quickly. Provided this is not so marked as to cause amnesia or disturb judgment, it can be a valuable asset, keeping the mind clear to tackle the next problem. Individuals less strongly endowed with this capacity can achieve the same result by deliberately diverting their minds (reading a book, digging in the garden) rather than sitting about dwelling on their difficulties.

4. The human help available. Whatever people may think about their self-knowledge, they rarely know themselves as well as they imagine. We need to learn about ourselves by feedback from parents, close relatives, best friends who *will* tell the truth. Because we change noticeably in our psychology every year or so throughout life, a feedback system is essential long after adolescence is past.

Close human relationships, as in marriage, for example, not only provide both partners with a better idea of their capabilities outside the home, but also help to combat stress by raising morale, clarifying situations, and rousing aggressiveness. Spontaneous remarks such as "Why do you let him get away with it," "Why should you always have to go to Washington," or "Forget it, he'll probably apologize on Monday," however simple they seem, not only comfort, but also protect the individual from a further sense of stress for a while.

Adaptation and Adjustment

Any person's effectiveness in adjusting to life can be readily appreciated by looking at the way he or she has adapted in three main areas of living. These are at work, in social life, and in sexual and family life. To these may be added religious life, which can make an important contribution to the other three.

In terms of the risk of breakdown, failure to adjust in one of these areas is unlikely to make the individual vulnerable, failure to adjust in two means greatly increased vulnerability, while failure in all three makes breakdown almost inevitable. Conversely, adjusting reasonably well in all three areas contributes not only to happiness but to the healthy state (probably chemically determined) of the nervous system on which all psychological activity is based. Consequently the presence of stress in one or more areas, unless resolved, decreases the person's chances of remaining healthy and happy.

It is relevant, however, to mention that stress in one area can be offset against greater satisfaction in another, at least for considerable periods. The opposite is also true—that neglect of the one area while another is promoted may lead to the former being lost. For example, an all too common experience is for a businessman who is bereaved to put all his efforts into business to help overcome the loss. Equally common is the man whose need to succeed and to conquer is satisfied at the expense of other areas of living. Family and friends are neglected and emotional relationships which are important enough on a daily basis are lost, and will be much mourned when it is too late.

OVERWORK AND CONFLICT

Of the three areas of living, work is the one in which stress is the most difficult to avoid. There is less option than in choosing one's friends or family. Even so, work is a very pleasant help when difficulties arise in other areas. Lack of work or of "belonging" in a work situation can be stressful in itself. Many people consider the nature of the work as a possible stress factor. This is unlikely to be the case in the practical or technical sense, and selection for the job usually ensures that employees have adequate skills. It is *people* who usually present the greatest problems. If a job is too difficult technically, changes can be made and the problem solved. Stresses are much greater in work requiring contact with others, as in selling, in jobs with much committee work, or jobs in which working in partnership or teams is the rule.

In the business field overwork is perhaps the most serious risk for the young executive. Its origins are clear enough, in that the desire to succeed is the predominant motivation of any person who takes on a job with a demanding workload, while there may also be a fear of failure arising partly from past failures, however minor these may have been.

In practical terms this conflict may lead to longer hours of work, fewer or increasingly unsociable hours at home, loss of sleep, alteration of habitual sleep patterns, irregularity of meals both in timing and in nature, and sacrifice of leisure time.

The development of this deviation from the generally accepted routine may be slow, but therein lies the danger. The slower the onset, the more easily is the burden accepted so that neither the worker nor his family protests firmly.

DANGER AHEAD!

Once a pattern of overwork has become established, risks are taken and certain secondary effects occur. The risks are of decreasing satisfaction from work and life generally as less compensatory time in social or leisure activity can be taken. Too little sleep or prolonged gross irregularity of sleep and meals can lead to a state of chronic tiredness, and lack of satisfaction in general, in which the individual forces himself, while functionally unfit, to complete the work while breaking down.

Chronic problems are more likely to persist when the demand for overtime comes not only from the office but from home as well. The sad but all too familiar story is of the man who works late or brings home work to improve his family's lot, but as this is being achieved the family raises its level of aspiration in terms of additional competition with the Joneses, thus forcing the breadwinner to stay on the treadmill. Other families increase the conflict (and risk of breakdown) by emphasizing the pleasures missed and outings canceled so that the conflict becomes more complex. In more direct form the conflicts can be illustrated as follows:

$$\text{Desire to succeed } versus \begin{cases} \text{fear of failure} \\ \text{fear of losing family} \end{cases}$$

As the effects of tiredness (or later depressive disorder) become apparent to the worker and to the employer the conflict is compounded further.

$$
\text{Desire to succeed } \textit{versus} \begin{cases} \text{fear of failure increased by:} \\ \text{actual failure} \\ \text{fear of losing job} \\ \text{fear of losing family} \end{cases}
$$

As the chances of succeeding fade so the individual's adjustment may suffer further.

CAUSES OF STRESS

While considering overwork, emphasis has been placed on the alteration of living rhythms forced on the individual. It cannot be overstated that it is these *imposed changes* which carry the penalty and not the extra hours of brain work involved. In the circumstances of business life, the strain of intellectual problem-solving is likely to prove difficult for long periods only as a result of monotony rather than true fatigue. Further confirmation of the importance of the alteration of life rhythms in causing ill health is provided by those few who break down after a period of disruption of their usual routine while producing in an artistic or creative sense their *magnum opus*. Every moment of the "work" has been enjoyable (it may even be a hobby) and the achievement of a masterpiece has brought its emotional reward, yet the symptoms of a depressive reaction can increase as the weeks pass even to the extent of incapacitating the artist and preventing completion of the work.

Where it is obvious to others that a person is overworking, the advice often offered is: "You have too much on your plate, why don't you give up this or that?" A very good question, but it is rarely necessary to ask it, for those who can jettison work or responsibility do so without being asked, and many who need to do so feel unable to.

There are two main patterns which lead to difficulty in relinquishing work and/or responsibility and an inability to delegate. One concerns the possession of that valuable obsessive trait of conscientiousness, the hallmark of the good citizen, but when developed to an unusual degree it forces the individual concerned not only to do his or her job well, but to ensure that it is perfect, checked to be perfect, and repeated if necessary to ensure that it is perfect. Such men and women may be unable to delegate because they fear that others' efforts will be incomplete or imperfect.

Another type with this sort of character experiences a painful sense of guilt if he is not over-employed; these people tend to impose on themselves (to the delight of a less sensitive employer) a workload to be compared in devotion to the task of the legendary bridge-painters who finally finish the job only to start repainting the same bridge the next day. Another common pattern associated with difficulty in delegating is a need for maintaining contact, and thereby power to influence others. If one does all the work in an important division employing twenty people, one is indeed indispensable and consequently powerful (and probably also very tiresome).

One futher pattern of behavior consists of spells of excessive activity followed by over-delegation with skimping of work, hurried project completion, and dissatisfaction among colleagues and co-workers.

Man in the Middle

A further source of conflict and tension among executives is their need to keep both their lords and masters and their juniors content while the motives and superficial aims of both may be in conflict. Anyone placed between two opposing forces in conflict cannot win all the time; the strain imposed may be reduced by a real acceptance of this fact. Fortunately, adjustment to changing circumstances by those above and below may lessen the pressures on the person in the middle and reduce the intensity of crises.

The position of the executive placed between higher management and the work force is often unenviable and difficult, but particularly so if the executive is handicapped by false perceptions. The forces inherent in the management/employee conflict can be readily magnified (and consequently mismanaged) by an unrealistic viewpoint taken by key personnel. Not only is the executive's sense of stress greater, but this may be reflected above and below, to the boardroom and the shop floor.

False perceptions are common enough in us all, though in some circumstances they can be helpful. Those with a sense of personal inferiority are hardest hit, in that they underestimate the respect paid them by seniors in the firm and magnify the adverse criticism from the juniors. Better communication could help the executive come to grips with the true position, but this is itself more difficult for individuals with such inferiority feelings, and this means of lessening their stress is often unused.

Over-Promotion, Underemployment And Job Frustration

Enthusiasm, intelligence, and drive can combine to thrust forward an ambitious individual too rapidly for his own or his colleagues' comfort. His greatest problems are likely to be concerned with personal relationships, and unless he is genuinely confident of his role various personal defense mechanisms may be necessary to protect him from feelings of inadequacy.

The behavior pattern which follows this is characteristically one of overcompensation, with tendencies to insist on excessive personal involvement in decision making, receiving praise or rewards, and stealing others' thunder. There is difficulty in the area of delegation; some over-delegate in a lordly fashion, whereas others cannot delegate sufficiently. Underemployment is not the paradise of which hard-working people dream. Overwork can harm health but (unfortunately for all our illusions) underemployment can do the same. If the three main areas of life satisfaction in mature people are reconsidered, there are few of us who can rely entirely on social life for enjoyment for long. Family life as a home-sweet-home concept may be delightful, but it is more important in the context of a base from which achievement in work, social life, and then marriage are made. Work satisfaction is usually the most important sector. There are many individuals without hobbies or interests of any kind. There are many who, sadly, neglect family and friends to give more time to their work, but there are very few well-adjusted and capable people who could do no work of any kind and remain fit and satisfied.

Although statistics need careful interpretation, it is interesting that the suicide rate declines during war or in times of economic health but increases during slumps. The reward from work is, of course, not merely financial: there is a social element, a sense of achievement, a sense of creation in some cases, and a sense of belonging to a team or providing a helpful service. A sense of responsibility or of power may be a factor.

The inactive state and its effects can readily be seen not only in those out of work but in those who are unable to get to work due to illness. Indeed, any doctor finds that unless patients are feeling extremely unwell it is often difficult to persuade them to remain inactive. Thirty years ago, when rest was essential for the recovery of tuberculous patients even when they felt physically and mentally fit, many found it impossible to observe the restrictions necessary over several months even though their lives were at stake.

So the need for work is strong and underemployment is a stress. It is biologically and psychologically healthier to help people to strive towards (and to achieve) a worthy goal than to give them too little to do.

Frustration in the course of the executive's work can arise in many ways: a sense of unfairness in the allocation of duties, getting the worst of rivalry between colleagues, or being taken advantage of as a "willing horse." More fundamental, however, is the stress imposed by a lack of feedback on results or an inability to identify with the aim of the firm. A subtle and frequently unrecognized aspect of job frustration occurs when pressures arising from an increased workload lead the executive to abandon the very parts of work which previously gave personal satisfaction. This may arise from a direct threat, so that the individual has no option but to struggle on with more strenuous chores or has to devote more time to maintaining a place in the power structure. Difficulties may arise when a policy change occurs due to economic necessity, or when there is a takeover.

Takeover Trauma

Takeovers provide the most dramatic and intense forms of stress for senior management and shop floor alike in the subdominant firm. The foundations of work satisfaction can be undermined while uncertainty about the future, doubts about new aims, deviation from traditional "safe" patterns of working, risk-taking and uncertainty about retaining the job itself—all of these contribute to anxiety, despondency, low morale, or even depressive illness.

Takeovers, with their power to control, to alter the pecking order, to remove prestige, to lower self-esteem and to cause losses in earnings and job satisfaction, involve much more strain and can lead to more repercussions than simple termination of employment. The emotional trauma is greatest when changes occur which affect those personnel closely identified with the firm, as in family businesses.

Personality Clashes

Personality clashes, a frequent source of tension at work, show infinite variety, yet there are some well-worn paths which can be avoided to prevent incompatibility. Any obvious disparities in intelligence, speed of thinking, talking, conscientiousness, selflessness, sociability, and background can be potential sources of strain. The central problem, however, that is likely to be met in business is the battle for power and prestige—the pecking order. In small organizations with a fairly rigid personnel structure the misfit's stay is unlikely to be prolonged; in larger firms where periodic selection determines the employee's future the battle for seniority is rarely confined to work achievement alone.

For the average executive there are certain patterns among colleagues likely to cause recurrent clashes. Then the relatively successful and well-adjusted person may start to blame himself for difficulties which he has neither encouraged, provoked, nor produced. This attitude may cause him to give in rather than fight, to his detriment and that of his firm.

Personality Types

Among the recurring personality types there is, first, the very markedly obsessive yet rigid individual who "stonewalls" himself throughout business (and social) life. A steady pace which cannot be varied, excessive concern with safety and routine hallowed by antiquity—these are his characteristics. Clashes occur from his inflexible attitudes, refusal to give and take, difficulty in working in teams and occasional passive but nevertheless aggressive postures, leading in extreme form to the attitude so well known now, and clearly described by Burton 350 years ago as: "like a hog or dog in the manger, he doth only keep it, because it shall do nobody else good, hurting himself and others."

Another striking figure is the larger-than-life human

dynamo whose character and temperament demand constant activity and grist for his mill. The pace here is fast and the road unending. Not infrequently such a person takes little sleep and apparently needs little. Difficulties arise because of the dynamo's refusal to accept the average person's slower (and often more precise) mode of thinking, working, or consolidating, and limitations in relation to energy output.

A grandiose attitude is sometimes associated with the strong drive of the human dynamo. The chief features are attitudes implying greater personal qualities than the individual in fact possesses. His conversation is punctuated with "I can do better" and a tendency to boast. His thinking is always towards the bigger achievements, the acquisition of status and a superior place with commensurate power. Colleagues resent the unjustified claims, unqualified opinions, pomposity, and presumptuousness of this type, but attempts to alter the situation frequently lead to aggression and abrasiveness on the part of the grandiose individual.

A very different picture is presented by the sensitive and precise personality whose feelings are easily hurt, yet whose determination demands that he or she should not be left out of the planning or decision-making. Others find imagined slights, apparently unaccountable aggression, and "heels dug in" attitudes exhausting yet inescapable. The attitude of such individuals can make them peevish and discontented, complainers for whom none can find a practical solution and none can escape blame.

The buck-passer is perhaps the hardest type to work with, for his or her principal belief is "it cannot be my fault, it must be yours." In more marked form it is the basis of the paranoid attitude.

Tensions in Teams and Groups
Other sources of frustration lie in the ways in which executives are held responsible and accountable for their

achievements or failures. Developments towards egalitarian management may lead to group situations producing high-intensity stress, whatever the terms of reference or details on the agenda. The basis of tension lies in the assumption that the contribution from each team member carries equal weight, wisdom, expertise, and authority. This assumption derives from a notion which is usually correct—that the representatives have equal power—but in practice the responsibility is not shared but is borne by one section of the group or occasionally by one individual. Difficulties usually arise when the "non-accountable to the project" members use delaying or other obstructive tactics for the sake of objectives unconnected with the goal itself. Since they have equal power, the ploy may be successful; with the result that the productivity of the group is poor, and those accountable are placed under excessive stress by uncertainty arising from a perpetually unpredictable outcome that has little to do with their real aims.

Such situations are compounded when individuals with vastly different qualifications have equal authority in the same team. Well-qualified executives may be overruled by a majority with unqualified opinions.

Travel Fatigue

Inseparable nowadays from the stressful scene of work is the stress of traveling to it, from it, and as part of business life itself (see Chapter 9). Few executives can live near their work, and the modern choice is between running an additional town apartment to make the office easily accessible, or going home to the family in the evenings with the twice-daily strain of traveling at peak hours.

Many people spend an hour a day driving a car, and this can in itself be a stressful experience. It is scarcely surprising that sudden illnesses can occur while people are driving, although relatively few accidents are due to illness. Driving can lead to an increase in the work of the heart, mainly shown by an increased heart rate in heavy traffic, poor driving conditions, and when there is a "near miss."

Despite the appalling conditions in which rush hour traveling takes place twice daily for millions, the effect on individuals is generally minimal. Adjustment takes place to the subway crush, standing in trains, lining up for buses or taxis and walking with armies of equally determined people along well-worn connecting routes. Stress does arise, however, when the routine level of discomfort is augmented by failure or uncertainty of services. The effects of strikes, job actions, power failures, severe weather conditions, and other inconveniences for the commuter are not only distressing and likely to induce anxiety, but their cumulative effect, involving alteration of life rhythms (an earlier start to the day, loss of sleep, no breakfast), anxiety about appointments or meetings, and when driving a car the fear of an accident, can lead to genuine illness.

Difficulties with Sleep

Insomnia is one of the most troublesome of complaints among executives, and its causes deserve analysis. Leaving aside the obvious causes of environmental noise and physical pain, there are two patterns which can be easily identified. The first (seen only in anxiety stress and certain varieties of depressive illness) is difficulty in falling asleep. It is generally the result of a failure to express feelings aroused during the day, leaving one alert and ready for appropriate action on retiring to bed, when these feelings no longer need to be suppressed. It can be due to unexpressed anger, unresolved anxiety, or unsolved problems of a threatening kind. But the basic problem is failure to act out feelings which have been generated but have not gained expression because of inhibiting circumstances at the time.

To a minor degree this tendency is seen in all those who read books or browse over magazines in bed to unwind before they go to sleep. It is often temporarily corrected by alcohol during the evening or by a stiff whisky nightcap; the real solution is usually obvious, yet frequently ignored. It is hardly necessary to add that if an executive in this state meets further tensions on arriving home, a tension debt can become impossible to redeem without a real change in lifestyle.

Another sleep disturbance seen in older people under stress is regular early morning waking. Although this is a hallmark of depressive illness, periods of early waking may herald the development of a full-blown illness, and the warning should be heeded. Typically the individual falls asleep without difficulty but finds himself waking up in the early hours, say between two and five a.m., worrying about the day ahead or work problems.

A distinction should be made between the subject's moods when early awakening occurs. The difference between waking in a state of concern, depression, dread, or anxiety, or with good spirits, plenty of energy, and plenty of constructive ideas is important. Whereas the former is reminiscent of depressive syndromes, the latter can precede phases of elation which, being most enjoyable for the person concerned, can develop into a condition of excessive excitement with disturbance of powers of judgment.

Planning for Retirement

Retirement these days may come earlier than before, as more and more emphasis is given to employing a younger, more energetic work force. Although many hard-working people may welcome the prospect of shedding the burden, the reality of retirement involves such vast changes that careful preparation is necessary.

After complete retirement there is a void where previously emotionally rewarding activity filled most of the day: a feeling that life is worth living has been lost, friends still busy in the firm are no longer met, a sense of belonging and being needed has been removed. Such changes can precipitate the well-known illness of post-retirement depression.

The health problems associated with aging add to the stress from the late fifties onwards. Although striking exceptions are seen, most people find their senses gradually failing, even in the absence of disease. Sight, hearing, smell, and taste decline slowly, and there is a gradual impairment of movement due to arthritis or muscular changes. This brings a realization not only of impairment, but also of a trend towards further deterioration. An unsatisfactory plan of retirement or a refusal to accept retirement may lead to disastrous results: the combined effect of loss of rewarding work and deterioration in health can mean severe suffering for the victim and his close relatives.

However, provided changes occur slowly enough, effective, healthy people of any age can and do adjust to retirement. Fortunately for them, executives are often better placed to make satisfactory arrangements for retirement than are members of other groups. In planning these changes, attention should be given to leisure and the development of hobbies. Friends should be made outside as well as inside the business, attention should be paid to health needs, and the financial situation should be fully worked out and secured. If possible, plans to continue one's participation in the firm on a part-time basis, or in an advisory capacity, should be arranged so that the loss of this very important area of satisfaction can be phased out slowly.

Lastly, although the element of stress in retirement has been emphasized there are many positive features. Giving up any burden can be a delight, and giving it up without guilt is positively exhilarating. There are ample opportunities to follow up hobbies and interests for which there was no time before. For a while social activities can be made more easily available, and the retired man or woman can contribute expertise or skills voluntarily to non-professional organizations rather than for financial reward. Although less dynamic, life can be a good deal more comfortable and secure.

The Executive's Spouse and Home

Home is in some ways a refuge from the stresses of work, but the ideal, so often entertained, of the pipe and slippers or the "friends in for drinks on the terrace" evening, is for many a fantasy. Nevertheless, the married man or woman has the potential for a less stressful lifestyle, and a successful marital relationship can sustain, energize, and comfort, maintaining a balance between the business jungle and the world outside.

As the home demands responsibilities, and the family grows and matures, their needs compete progressively with the demands of the office. As already described, the scene is set for conflict, affection and loyalty to family competing with the fear of falling down on the job or failing to compete successfully when the next opportunity for advance arises. Unless the worker is able to manage this conflict successfully, his or her investment in time at work is likely not only to deprive the spouse and immediate family but also to weaken family friendships and the family's social life.

At this point it can be seen that a situation may arise in which stress directed at the executive can be passed on to the spouse and children. How far this occurs is an individual matter. How far it repercusses to impose compound stress on the executive depends on the family's aims and strengths and on the marital relationship itself. For this reason, it is necessary to consider the stresses felt by wives and the possible outcome of excessive stress in this direction.

Margaret L. Helfrich, in a United States' study titled *The Social Role of the Executive Wife,* discusses such questions as "Why has the wife of an executive become so important?" She studied fifty wives, and the consensus view of their roles was (1) to take care of the home and children, (2) to manage so that time could be found for the husband,

(3) to keep the income running smoothly and to be able to entertain, and (4) to participate to some extent in civic and social affairs.

J. M. and R. E. Pahl in a British study found managers' wives occasionally having difficulty in being objective about themselves and their roles. Helfrich found that a typical wife was generally less interested in the work situation than in her husband's work as he expressed it, and as she experienced it in terms of the demands of the job, the status achieved, and the financial rewards. While welcoming the material advantages and the satisfaction it gave to their husbands, many wives felt a degree of antagonism towards the husband's firm, resenting the long hours of work or absences from home the job entailed and the inevitable conflict between the husband's work and family roles.

In a good marriage the relationship between husband and wife is sufficiently close and strong to allow considerable flexibility in the husband's work schedule. In the early days the wife is usually inexperienced at entertaining and finds it more of a strain, but there is usually less entertaining to do. It can become difficult to manage the children and find time for the social demands of the husband's business.

In the ideal situation, however, the most successful executive will gain more time with his family as promotion and movement within the business structure allows this, and his wife will be expected to do more entertaining only during that period when the children are growing up. Reality compromises this ideal, but the more it does so, the greater the mutual strain and risk of marriage failure. To avoid this it is essential that family and domestic problems of any importance should be shared, discussed, faced together, and where possible resolved. Time has to be given to the growing children's needs by both parents, for not only is any deficiency here difficult or impossible to remedy later, but any problems which arise during adolescence or early adult life will be far more time-consuming.

When the Wife Is the Executive

Married female executives always have two jobs. Both are time-consuming and demanding, and unless a continuous compromise is arranged, conflict is inevitable. The conflict between efficiency in the office and the time, thought, and affection needed by husband and children regularly recurs, for both need daily attention. Even weekends can be encumbered by business writing and planning. The time that has to be found for the demands of husband and children is often unpredictable in nature and degree, and if time is short and energy limited, the schedule carefully planned to satisfy all needs is often disrupted and frustrates everyone involved. The problems encountered specifically by women deserve a chapter to themselves (see Chapter 4).

PATTERNS OF STRESS

At this point the different patterns produced by stress can be considered. The average person often thinks of headache or ulcer pain as a sign of stress, when these may well be purely physical problems caused by eye strain or gastritis. In practice, any symptom can arise from stress, and it is probable that the pattern of symptoms shown is related to the personality of the sufferer. Although it is not possible to give a comprehensive account of this relationship, a broad impression can be given.

Individuals can be considered to have various personality traits in varying proportions, and it is only when certain of these traits are predominant, present in strength and not balanced by other traits, that the personality can be described in this or that way. The main personality types we are concerned with in the business world are:

1. The obsessive personalities, who tend to be reliable, conscientious, dependable, predictable and to suppress expression of emotional feelings. They prefer routine

45

and a conservative approach, and the traits of good citizenship are well marked.

2. The sensitive personalities, who tend to be much more sensitive than average to other people's feelings and opinions and to atmosphere generally. They attune themselves more rapidly and are better able to understand others' difficulties. They can become emotionally involved more easily and tend to be more suggestible and introverted. Emotional feelings are more readily expressed; many earn the description of being "natural."

3. The combination of certain obsessive and sensitive traits in the same individual is particularly common in the general population, in both work force and management. Sensitivity to people, situations, audiences, and atmosphere is coupled with characteristic emotional inhibition. Whereas the person concerned is easily aroused emotionally, he or she keeps a stiff upper lip, and feelings remain bottled up. This tendency is variable, and the majority of the population find outlets of a socially acceptable kind. It is when these outlets are poor that an individual may be vulnerable to the stress described.

The effects of stress depend on whether the change is of the sudden, overwhelming variety or a chronic unsolved conflict, and it is necessary to consider both types of stress for each personality type.

Considering first the effects of sudden overwhelming stress, the obsessive person shows little outward signs of distress. He or she may occasionally feel a temporary weakness or emotional numbness, but carries on with work and other duties with little deviation.

In contrast, the sensitive individual reacts quickly and freely and tends to express all the intense feelings likely to be engendered by an emotional shock of this kind. The well-known signs of emotional upset appear, including tears, rapid and sometimes incoherent speech, and occasionally "hysterics." In some cases temporary hysterical conversion symptoms such as loss of voice, a lump in the throat, or spasm of muscles around the eyes may be precipitated.

Those with obsessive and sensitive traits under these conditions tend to be anxious, tremulous, or tearful. Others become tense, and a few develop transient nervous rash.

The effects of, second, a chronic conflict of unremitting emotional overload can produce a state of lasting tension in the obsessive individual. Later a depressive illness or anxiety state may ensue. The sensitive person is vulnerable to the development of hysterical conversion symptoms, and these are more likely to persist until the stress lifts. In a chronic situation these symptoms are more profound and can include loss of use of a limb or loss of sight. Depressive illness may also develop in this personality type. Those with both sensitive and obsessional features also tend to develop either depressive reactions, anxiety states, or chronic psychosomatic conditions.

DEPRESSIVE ILLNESSES AND THEIR EFFECTS

Depressive illness probably affects one in fifteen of the population at some time and its nature is often misunderstood. The illness has different characteristics in the young and in older subjects.

The typical depression seen in older, obsessive people is characterized by tiredness, lack of drive, finding everything an effort, and feeling worse in the mornings and better as the day wears on. Sleep is disturbed by early morning waking, often with a sense of dread. Appetite, weight, and sexual drive are reduced. There is a lack of initiative, a tendency to worry about trivia, a gloomy outlook which disturbs judgment, and a loss of normal aggressiveness. There is a tendency to drink more alcohol and to smoke more heavily.

The change in outlook and tendency to become pre-occupied with gloomy outcomes can affect business judgments. Think of the situation as two sides of a coin. The depressive patient looks at the negative side which produces feelings of unworthiness, hopelessness, remembrance of past failure, coupled with dread of future disaster and catastrophic outcome. It is probable that these experiences and thoughts moved into the "memory store" according to the tone attached to events at the time. The other side of this coin will have stored up pleasant, positive, useful, and encouraging thoughts.

Most healthy people view this hypothetical storage system askew, in that they focus on the positive, useful memories and their past successes and future ambitions, wearing as it were rose-tinted glasses. In this way the scene (and mind) is set for decision, initiative, and progress. In depressive illness, however, the viewpoint shifts to the unhappy side so that the same individual is now constantly preoccupied with gloomy thoughts of future hopelessness. Decisions become difficult because all future forecasts are now tinged with the prospect of disaster, and the unfortunate sufferer is faced with the choice between Scylla and Charybdis throughout the day, day after day. This indecisiveness is only one effect of the illness, but it is of great importance in slowing down the individual's output and rendering him incapable of true leadership.

A typical depression seen in younger and more sensitive individuals is characterized by difficulty in getting to sleep, a tendency to increased appetite, weight, and sexual drive with worsening of the symptoms of fatigue, irritability, aggressiveness, and tension in the afternoons and evenings.

Fortunately these illnesses have an excellent prognosis with treatment, and once the individual has recovered there is no impairment of psychological integrity. It is worth repeating here that such illnesses are not necessarily a result of work difficulty, although to the sick patient work becomes an intolerable burden and may be blamed. There are many other precipitants, from unexpressed grief or anger, the effects of certain drugs including alcohol, and aftereffects of severe infections or surgical operations, to the effects of hormones, including in some women the contraceptive pill. It is important to consider such possibilities carefully before reducing the level of responsibility of someone who may have spent much of his life attaining a position that, with help, he is still capable of fulfilling.

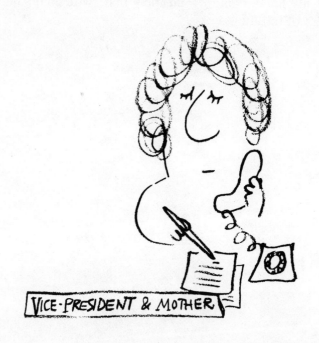

VICE-PRESIDENT & MOTHER

chapter 4

WOMEN AT WORK

Throughout the book you will read of the general problems of stress for the executive; it is no longer easy to assume that the executive is invariably male. This is undoubtedly not true today, and it will become even less true in the future. More and more women have professions, and more of them are choosing to stay at work throughout their working life.

When it comes to stress, what applies to men also applies to women—but more so. I do not mean the extra pressures for a woman trying to climb the executive ladder against possible male (and female) prejudice; the pressure I am referring to is that of trying to do two jobs at once. Working all day and then starting again in the evening is bound to add to the normal stresses of executive life. As a senior executive on a daily newspaper, I have seen surprisingly little of the effects of stress which can lead to illness; nor have I noted it affecting women executives more than men. Nervous breakdowns seem to be distributed with more regard to personality than to sex. It is true to say, however, that few women so far have scaled the executive heights as far as the summit, so it is too soon to compare their responses to stress with their male colleagues.

There are a few statistical straws in the wind to suggest that the diseases which have traditionally attacked the male who is working outside the home are beginning to attack women as well. Certainly, many more women are picking up bad habits: the trend in smoking among women is still rising, and they are reported to be drinking more and swelling the ranks of alcoholics.

But stress is stress, wherever it appears. Young women isolated in high-rise apartment buildings all day with small children have shown signs of severe stress. The breakup of the extended family seems to have had a similar result. Domestic stress can be as severe as that at work. The problem probably arises most among women who—if you like—want to have the best of everything. Those who want good jobs and want to rise on the executive ladder, but who also want normal families, are painfully aware that society expects of them a further role—that of looking after their husbands and their children.

THE WORKING WIFE

It seems sensible to look first at the stresses which can arise for a married woman who tries to continue her traditional role as well as working. She knows that if anything goes wrong in the home and she is not there, she will be blamed because she goes out to work. Outlandish claims are sometimes made that the children of women who have jobs outside the home make slower progress at school and that they form the biggest proportion of juvenile delinquents. Such suggestions do not stand up to rigorous study; the underlying factors throughout seem to be both material and emotional deprivation. The physical absence of the mother for part of the time seems to be unimportant as long as a child has some supervision and constant attention. Unfounded suggestions, however, that a child will not develop properly into a mature and balanced adult if its mother works can put great stress on the working mother.

The truth is that a mother can often build up a better long-term relationship with her children if she has worked than if she has not. Children can become too accustomed to their mother's presence, taking her for granted and largely ignoring her, while being with their father remains a special treat. Working women can also be treats, if their time with their children is rationed. They are likely to take more positive pleasure in being with the children more, too.

Children who are left a little to their own resources tend to be independent and healthy. (Teacher to my daughter: "Why is it that you are *never* ill?" Child: "In our house we are only ill on Saturdays and Sundays.") It is astonishing how healthy the children of working women seem to be. Petty aches and pains are rushed off to school, invariably vanishing on the way. Of course the children of working mothers have the same needs as those whose mothers do not work, but those needs are love and security, and neither depends on the constant presence of the mother in the house.

For many couples today marriage is no longer a hier-archical institution, with the man at the head leading his wife and children. More and more couples are finding that a genuine partnership is more rewarding for both of them. Difficulties are more likely to arise for a woman with a husband who feels that he has no responsibilities at home; she will probably find it extremely difficult to lead a working life of any kind, and almost impossible to carry out an executive function in a com-pany. Fortunately, it seems that many women who do want a life outside their home instinctively choose the more caring and cooperative men, who are prepared to participate in running the home and to respect their wife's career demands.

Before a woman sets out on the executive trail she should carefully consider the implications. They are fairly straight-forward, but can bring severe stress if not tackled properly. She should work out what the job involves and assess whether she can do it properly and reliably, given the other demands made upon her. She should discuss the matter fully with her husband, and be sure of his cooperation and support—and his willingness to take on some of the family chores. She should also ask herself whether she really wants to work, whether the fullfill-ment of having a career will compensate for the extra demands on her time and energy.

Women in positions of responsibility must accept that they cannot do two jobs. There should be no attempt to try to do all the cleaning, ironing, and so forth for the family as well as a demanding job outside the home. Those responsibilities must go elsewhere, though there is of course no reason why some of the more enjoyable tasks—such as cooking the family dinner—should not be undertaken or shared. The family should learn to participate too, by helping to prepare the meal, to serve and to wash up.

The demands of the job may sometimes have to come before those of the family; a working mother with small chil-dren must *completely* replace herself at home, as odd hours, mornings, or days cannot be taken from an executive position. If she hopes for promotion, a woman at work must be considered as reliable as a man in the same position. It costs a good deal of money to replace oneself at home. Children work as hard at school as an adult does in a job, and there is a limit to the amount of help they should be expected to give. A reliable, well-paid cleaner is therefore essential to take care of all the more mundane aspects of running a home. The executive woman must ensure that when she is at home her husband and family get her attention, and that they can sit down together and relax in the evening. A mother who is ironing while the other members of her family talk, watch television, or take part in games is depriving them of her attention when they need it. They do not need it when they are at work or school, so she must be available at the time she is wanted—just as a father should be. The mother's replacement must be reliable, because a woman executive cannot take time off, any more than a man could, if a child is sick or on school holidays.

STRESS AND THE SINGLE WOMAN

The stresses faced by married people are quite different from those faced by the single, and single career women have a problem which does not always face the single man. Some women undoubtedly feel that they have to give up any opportunity of family life if they are to succeed in their career—and the number of divorces among career women tends to support this view to some extent. Looking around at their male colleagues, women recognize that no such basic choice is involved for men. This is not to say, of course, that men never sacrifice their marriages for their careers—though they tend not to move into celibate lives, but rather to live in a situation of continuous monogamy with a series of wives, ensuring that the basic patterns of their lives are not disturbed. Many single career women will choose to have a series of relationships rather than the demands of a husband and family. But some career women see no such option. If they succeed in their chosen careers, no stress or regret may enter their lives, but if they have not been too successful they may well feel (often when their childbearing days are over) that the sacrifice of a family has been too great.

STRESS IN THE OFFICE

When it comes to the office and promotion, women tend to find two things against them. The first is their biology and the myths surrounding it; the second to some extent follows from the first. They may face the prejudice of the male colleagues and, even worse, the resentment of other women who may not do so well in their jobs.

It is hardly possible to open a newspaper today without reading of the problems of menstruation or the menopause. It is a fact that all women menstruate and all women eventually go through the menopause. Suggestions that they may be less efficient on "certain days" or at a "certain age" plague most women as they go through their careers. This attitude can easily induce the very symptoms they are alleged to have. A woman who rightly loses her temper is regarded as "hysterical," while a man is just "angry"; a firm woman executive is "bossy," a man simply "decisive." There are many similar descriptions which illustrate this point. Many people are not yet accustomed to women being in executive positions and there are still residual feelings that their *only* place is in the home (especially in a time of unemployment)—that by working they do men out of jobs. There may also be resentment from some people simply because when they were small their mothers represented the voice of authority and were therefore to be rebelled against.

Men are used to being dominant, and often carry their behavior in the family with them to work. Pity, then, the poor woman executive, who may find she is expected to fetch and carry for men with whom she is theoretically on the same executive level, but who take it for granted that women are there to carry on where their wives leave off! (I am not just carping. I have had a senior editorial job for ten years now, and from time to time men still come and ask me if I would mind doing a bit of typing for them. Fortunately I made sure early on that I would never be able to type well).

A woman executive is still newsworthy.[1] How many male bank managers are regarded as worthy of a story in the national press, for example? This relative rarity means that they are likely to be more scrutinized than their male counterparts, that mistakes they make will be regarded more seriously, and that they will be required to demonstrate their abilities in a far more obvious way than a man. It would be foolish to deny, however, that men and women can work together on an equal basis, and it is an idea that should increasingly become accepted.

Nevertheless, the old myths die hard, and they can be extremely difficult to live and work with. Few women executives can have lived out their careers without encountering one of the following myths: women are too emotional and illogical to be good at business; a woman's children are damaged for life if she goes out to work; any woman who does not particularly want a husband or children is unnatural; women do not have the ruthless streak necessary for a good executive career; women are too ruthless; women who go out to work are unfeminine; women use their sex to get their own way; women are ineffective for a considerable part of the month because of premenstrual tension; women's biology limits their ambitions;

---

[1] For a further analysis of this visibility problem see *In the Spotlight: Women Executives in a Changing Environment,* Margaret Fenn, © 1980 Prentice-Hall, Inc.

women take too much time off work looking after their children; a woman boss is a contradiction in terms.

Of course many of these myths are contradictory, but
they can be disturbing and lead to stress. Any woman who has
worked in an executive role for some years knows that they are
nonsense; nevertheless, the constant taunts in themselves create
stress—so much so, that some women in the end accept them
as the truth and abandon their ambitions. Others learn to live
with them. But it takes time and even after many years it may
be difficult not to react with hostility.

The only way out for women is not to react. There is
nothing wrong in being a woman who chooses to work in a
competitive world alongside men. There is nothing wrong
with a woman combining parenthood with having a career—
millions of men do it. There is nothing wrong with a woman
choosing a career rather than a family. Finally, there is nothing
wrong with a woman developing her personality in the way
she wishes. Women, like men, only live once and must make
the best of their resources in their own way. They don't get
a second chance.

This is good for me..
This is (puff) good for (puff) my heart..
This (puff) is (puff) good.. (puff)..

chapter 5

TAKE HEART

In the early years of this century doctors and nurses knew a great deal about making the best of an individual's health if it proved to be inadequate for his needs and deteriorated from overloading. Attitudes changed after the last war as people learned of the wonderful effects of new drugs such as antibiotics. Tuberculosis, for example, could be cured without the need for prolonged residence in a sanatorium, and pneumonia no longer required careful nursing and an anxious wait for the crisis to pass.

Naturally enough, people sought this sort of cure for all their ailments, and physicians, too, became more dependent upon drug treatments. As the doctors tried harder to satisfy the demands of the public they became more and more involved with the chemical and physical processes inside the body and paid less heed to the behavior and circumstances of the patient.

Unfortunately for this trend in medicine, our behavior and circumstances cannot be put aside. These factors have a great deal to do with our losing the ability to cope, becoming ill, and breaking down. The chemical and physical processes inside the body are sensitive to the ways in which life is lived, but they have only a limited capacity for remaining normal. Drug therapy can be irrelevant and harmful where the lifestyle is straining these chemical and physical processes beyond their tolerance.

It is, for example, quite natural for a man's blood pressure to be raised by prolonged periods of exhausting hard work, particularly if he smells defeat in the air, and his relationship with his wife may be disturbed by business preoccupations. If he does not take a period of rest and relaxation, to compensate for the hard period and to allow his blood pressure to fall to normal again, but asks for a drug to bring down his blood pressure, he may be given drugs which, as an unfortunate side effect, reduce his capacity for sexual intercourse. This, in turn, reduces his confidence and aggression, aggravates his marital problems, and teaches him nothing about adopting working

59

methods which neither exhaust the mind nor inflict hypertension upon the heart and arteries.

These observations are of particular importance in malfunction of the heart and arteries, where small changes in behavior and circumstances help to make the most of the individual's health. When the emphasis is put on behavior the patient learns that he or she is to be responsible for halting deterioration and initiating improvement: the physician's role is that of trainer and technical adviser. This is quite a different matter from the patient adopting a passive role in a relationship with the physician, or being weakly submissive when little understood things are done by a hospital that has become a technical workshop.

What advice, then, can be given to the executives who fear that they may be living or working dangerously in an urban world or business hierarchy and wish to keep their hearts and arteries in the best possible condition for healthy function? First, a low priority should be given to drugs and dietary measures; these treatments have already been the subject of overwhelming propaganda that may prove to have little relationship to the truth. Instead, the prevention and treatment of heart disorders should be based on a clear understanding of the effects of behavior on health.

HEART AILMENTS

The function of the heart can be disturbed in a variety of ways. It can lack *power,* either because it is not trained for the job in hand or because it has suffered a temporary or permanent injury. Its *rhythm* can become too fast, too slow, or irregular, and these changes of rhythm may also be temporary or permanent. The human response to the symptoms or feelings produced by these disturbances of function is immensely varied. Some individuals are insensitive to their inner workings and may be unconscious of any disturbance until the point of breakdown is reached; others are easily upset by quite small departures from normal. It has nothing to do with strength of character or endurance—some individuals capable of the highest flights of human performance show a keen awareness of fluctuations in the health upon which their fortunes depend.

The pumping equipment of the heart may be abnormal at birth from hereditary causes or maternal illness during pregnancy. Later in life the heart structure can be injured by a wide range of natural causes including rheumatism, infectious diseases, vitamin deficiencies, alcoholism, and chronic respiratory disease; and its functions can be disturbed by such conditions as anemia and diseases of the thyroid gland. These conditions are rare in men and women leading active, busy lives; for all practical purposes their risk is from the heart attacks and strokes which are caused by disorders of the vital arteries feeding the heart (the coronary arteries) and the brain (the cerebral vessels). Attacks of illness from these kinds of arterial disease are so common in Western urban life that they are often assumed to be determined by fate. In fact, individual behavior has a profound influence on coronary ill health and heart attacks.

THE HUMAN FUNCTION CURVE

The easiest way to understand these important relationships between behavior and health is through the concept of the human function curve. If arousal—stimulation from external events and inward striving—is plotted against performance—the ability to cope with tasks—the graph shows the natural changes in behavior that lead from health to breakdown. In a healthy individual, increasing the arousal increases the performance. The gain falls off in fatigue. Once someone is exhausted, however, persistence of the arousal causes the actual

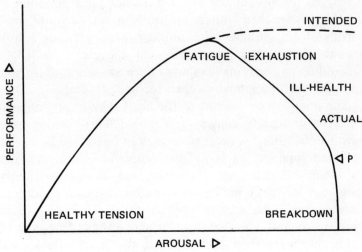

Human Function Curve

performance to deteriorate and fall below the intended level. If there is no relief from the arousal the exhaustion gives way to ill health. Eventually a point (P) is reached where little further arousal is required to precipitate a breakdown or catastrophe.

It does not take a doctor's training to recognize these aspects of human behavior. Every administrator should be aware of them.

RECOGNITION OF HEALTHY FUNCTION

Someone who is healthy feels well. The manner is relaxed, and physical recreation brings pleasure. The idea of spending time relaxing and taking exercise does not cause guilty reactions. Burdens and pressures that would cause loss of happiness and health are rejected. The qualities required for success—rapid and flexible thought, originality, vigor, expansion, and capacity for sustained effort—are all obvious to other people.

Such an individual feels and accepts reasonable fatigue, does not deny it, and takes steps to recover as soon as possible. He realizes that habits that waste time and energy can be modified and inessential drains on the energy can be jettisoned or deferred. In fatigue, performance can increase with arousal but more effort is required. Disciplined effort, youthful conditioning for competition, social pressures, and mild stimulants such as coffee and cigarettes, all play a greater part in sustaining the performance. Sleep is adequate. Others see the individual as healthily tired, but they are not made anxious because the qualities required for success are still evident. Therapy is neither sought nor required, though reassurance that the fatigue is healthy may be sought by volunteers for checkups.

EXHAUSTION

Exhaustion of the individual's ability to cope with the demands he places upon himself (or accepts from others) has a wide range of effects on his own life and on those around him. Few people realize how easily reversible the condition can be, and most accept it as a "normal" way of life. The characteristic feature of exhaustion is that the harder the individual pushes himself (or allows himself to be pushed by others) the worse his performance becomes. This vicious circle operates against him as his declining ability to cope generates more arousal which, in turn, causes further deterioration in performance. Heightened arousal interferes with sleep, further aggravating the exhaustion. Anxiety and guilt increase arousal further. Previously acceptable and useful characteristics become unbalanced, encourage inefficiency, and disrupt the peace of mind of others.

For example, the careful manager may become obsessed with detail, pedantic, and incapable of delegating responsibility. Bad temper and inappropriately aggressive behavior increase the problems at work and at home. The ability to discriminate between essential and inessential matters is easily lost when an individual is under pressure, and long-term aims may be lost to sight in an exasperating preoccupation with petty matters. Longer hours are worked, but less is achieved. Noncommunicative verbiage replaces crisp commands. Job satisfaction and self-esteem wane. Complaints of frustration or persecution by others come to the fore. Leadership comes to depend upon rank and seniority and not upon a greater enjoyment of the qualities required for success.

Once in this state an exhausted executive commonly makes strong declarations of health and ability that are at odds with observed behavior. He or she rejects the need to maintain a healthy balance between high endeavor and relaxation and sees no need to increase physical fitness in preparation for periods of intensive effort, becoming unfit and inactive. Sometimes he or she puts spurts of effort into physical activity in the mistaken belief that exercise can cure the disorders of exhaustion.

Physical Changes

Changes in the internal chemical environment of the body develop in response to the exhaustion caused by prolonged and excessive arousal. These include increases in the heart rate and blood pressure and in the blood fats (cholesterol and triglycerides are the most commonly tested), uric acid, sugar, and coagulability. These changes are mostly due to overactivity of the sympathetic nervous system and the action of hormones such as the catecholamines (adrenalin and noradrenalin) and ACTH which stimulate the adrenal cortex. The hormonal response to arousal is, in fact, a normal function of the brain developed by evolution. It is the natural mechanism for meeting physical challenges—either fighting or running away—for involvement in the pecking order of an organization, and for the display of appeasement maneuvers. These brain functions are also profoundly affected by those overwhelming life situations which deprive the individual of the choice of any acceptable course of action.

Other changes in the internal chemistry are produced by the characteristic tendency of the exhausted to eat, drink, and smoke too much. Swelling of the legs from an accumulation of fluid is especially common in women. Pains in the chest, palpitations, sensations of breathlessness, and feelings of discomfort related to the heart all occur and may be accompanied by air swallowing, gaseous distention of the stomach, and belching. Assurance by a doctor that no signs of disease can be found usually provides little more than temporary relief because the patient *knows* that he or she is not functioning well.

Attempts to bring about an improvement often make the spouse and the doctor frustrated and tense because the more severe the patient's exhaustion the more seriously attempts to reduce arousal are resisted: duty, loyalty, righteous indignation, militant enthusiasm, and a compulsive desire for excitement are commonly used devices, and these may carry the exhaustion on into ill health. And yet exhaustion is the worst condition to be in when survival depends upon the human qualities required for success.

Psychological Responses

The average executive's inability to recognize and deal with exhaustion has several explanations. If changes are seen at all they might be regarded as the irremediable defects of aging and the executive may fight to overcome them—the one measure guaranteed to make conditions worse and to create a self-defeating depression. More often the psychological maneuver of "denial" takes over to veil the deterioration that cannot be faced, and so there seems to be no need for action. A second psychological maneuver of "projection" sometimes moves in to shift the blame for deterioration and the responsibility for action on to the shoulders of others. Thirdly, the "displacement" maneuver can cause the individual to be too busy and preoccupied with trivia to stand back and survey the position objectively. If the symptoms are obscured by denial maneuvers or if they are erroneously dismissed as the effect of aging, the signs of ill health may be revealed at a routine medical examination or one made at the request of a relative or colleague. Diagnosis depends upon the doctor knowing enough about the patient to recognize the pre-existing exhaustion—and having enough experience of life to recognize that the patient's circumstances have been difficult enough for long enough to produce the threat of ill health. Recovery depends on treating the exhaustion and excessive arousal and not on remedies prescribed to remove symptoms. This principle applies to prestigious remedies, such as heart operations for angina, just as much as to the use of simple painkillers for headaches.

Illnesses Associated with Exhaustion

Many types of ill health may be brought about by long continued exhaustion and arousal. Some individuals run true to form and find themselves carried off the field of battle by the same sort of illness every time they overstretch their resources. Others fall ill with a wider variety of disorders. The differences are probably related to age and sex, inherited characteristics, family influences in early life, the amount of arterial wear and tear already present, and the quality of support provided by others.

The general practitioner may see patients suffering from infectious diseases because their powers of resistance are lowered, or from accidents because their minds are preoccupied. Aches and pains related to the muscles, joints, backs, and discs are especially common. The heart specialist sees patients suffer-

ing predominantly from the biochemical and structural consequences of high and prolonged arousal. These include high
blood pressure; gout from raised blood uric acid levels; venous
thrombosis and embolism from increased blood coagulability
(Richard Nixon after Watergate); abnormal blood levels of
cholesterol and the triglycerides; and various forms of painful
(*angina pectoris*) or painless cardiac dysfunction.

Some individuals are incredibly tough and can continue
to function in the zones of exhaustion and ill health until they
run out of strength or suffer a breakdown from a chance ag-
gregation of adverse circumstances. In urban societies throughout the world it is increasingly common for the breakdown to
take the form of a heart attack, or coronary.

CORONARY BREAKDOWN

As long ago as 1908 Sir James Mackenzie pointed out that
heart patients rarely sought treatment until some distressing
symptom interrupted the course of their lives. He described
the four varieties of breakdown that are now called acute left
ventricular failure, acute coronary insufficiency, myocardial
infarction, and sudden death from a heart attack.

The left ventricle is the main pumping chamber of the
heart, responsible for driving the blood into the aorta with
sufficient force to carry it through the arteries and capillaries
into the venous return side of the circulation. Failure of the
left ventricle has two consequences: not enough blood is driven
forward to meet the needs of the body, and too much is dammed
back in the lungs. The results are great weakness and great
breathlessness. The causes of the failure include the sudden
throwing of too great an emotional or physical burden upon
an unprepared heart, perhaps by raising the blood pressure
abruptly, and any one of the disorders of the heartbeat which

make the pumping action too quick or too slow. Failure occurs more readily when the coronary arteries are narrowed.

Acute coronary insufficiency is a malfunction of the left ventricle suffering from a sudden drop in its supply of oxygen and nutrients in the blood. This occurs when the demands put upon pumping action exceed the ability of the coronary arteries to channel blood to the heart muscle. Obviously it is easier for the demands to exceed the supply when the arteries are narrowed by disease. Acute coronary insufficiency is one cause of a heart attack—the sudden onset of crushing pain in the chest, often associated with collapse, sweating, and profound weakness. It may also disturb the nerve centers and the electrical conducting system that regulates the heart beat, and the pumping action may be arrested—switched off. If the heartbeat is stopped for more than a few minutes death ensues. Prompt first-aid treatment with cardiac massage can keep the circulation going until the heartbeat is restored even when the cardiac arrest has taken place in the street. The occurrence of acute coronary insufficiency and cardiac arrest do not necessarily imply that the heart has run out of its natural life span. They may be accidental in the sense that a successfully treated patient can lead a normal life afterwards.

Myocardial infarction is the term used to describe a condition of permanent damage to the heart muscle caused by a lack of blood supply. The amount of damage can range from slight to catastrophic. The infarction can occur in people with apparently normal coronary arteries, but it is easier for high and prolonged arousal to drive a man from ill health to myocardial infarction when the arteries are narrowed.

Sudden death from a heart attack can result from electrical disorders in acute coronary insufficiency and myocardial infarction or from overwhelming damage to the pumping mechanism. Again, it is more easily brought about when the arteries are severely narrowed.

ARTERIAL DISEASE

It is important to keep a sense of proportion about coronary artery disease. A coronary breakdown may be brought about more easily when the narrowings are severe, but the arteries of active men killed accidentally in old age often look worse than those of young men who die of a heart attack. And middle-aged men with severe narrowings of the three major coronary arteries can be trained to become marathon runners. With nature offering resources such as these it is unnecessary for someone found to have arterial disease to give way to gloom and pessimism.

Narrowing of the coronary arteries is caused by damage to their lining from a fatty deposit, atheroma. Three major abnormalities are common precursors. First, if the blood pressure is raised the lining may be damaged and fatty material forced through the lining into the arterial wall. The second factor is an increase in the amount of fatty compounds in the bloodstream—the raised levels of cholesterol and triglycerides. The third is an increased stickiness of the blood platelets, which clump together where the lining is damaged and encourage the formation of a thrombus or clot.

Medical opinion has not yet agreed about either the details of these processes or their relative importance. Nor has it agreed about the best ways of slowing down atheromatous damage—and since there seems little prospect of early agreement we must make the best of what we know.

As long ago as the nineteenth century it was known that when the hormone adrenalin was given to rabbits for several weeks the aorta became atheromatous. More recently human research has shown that prolonged stress can raise blood pressure and provoke heart disease. The behavioral and environmental associations of heart attacks conform to the same pattern.

These research findings are important because they lay a foundation for optimism by providing a rational plan for the management of the hypertension—atheroma—heart disease problem. The three major factors that provoke atheroma formation can be controlled by the individual to a remarkable degree, and so can the subsidiary factors—cigarette smoking, which increases noradrenalin activity, and obesity and unfitness, which appear to encourage the production of cholesterol and triglycerides. An excess of carbohydrates in the diet (or an inability to process them adequately, as in diabetes) may also encourage the cholesterol and triglycerides to rise above a healthy level when the forces of hyperarousal and exhaustion are at work. However, these subsidiaries have a relatively small part to play.

In 1958 Friedman, Rosenman, and Carroll reported that the cholesterol level and blood coagulability of accountants varied according to their "stresses": one of their patients had a cholesterol level of 326 mgm percent when under extreme pressure and 231 mgm percent when on holiday. Most patients with raised blood cholesterol and triglyceride concentrations respond to the reduction of arousal and the relief of exhaustion.

On the other hand, the evidence does not yet justify the current emphasis on the amount of fat in the diet. It would, indeed, be odd if natural meat and dairy products had become poisonous to man in the twentieth century. We would not have evolved as man with feet for walking and hands for grasping if we had not been able to obtain most of our structural fat and energy requirement from animals. In 1975 Lord Taylor looked at the distribution of coronary heart disease in the United Kingdom. It is not more prevalent in the relatively affluent southeast, and it does not follow the pattern for lung cancer—as it might if cigarettes were a major cause. The areas of highest mortality are those of most recent emergence from poverty.

Cigarette-smoking is said to be an important coronary risk factor by most advisers on health. There are, however, some objections to giving it a major role. Without a doubt, some individuals have uncommonly powerful responses to the effects of cigarette smoking which easily put up their blood pressure, blood cholesterol and triglycerides, and blood co-agulability: these sensitive people have a better than average reason for giving up. There is also, of course, the proven association between smoking and lung cancer—in itself a good enough reason for any rational individual to become a nonsmoker.

An excessive use of coffee has been associated with hypertension and heart disease. If such a relationship exists it is probably because coffee makes it easier for the exhausted work-addict to keep working to the point of breakdown.

Moderate degrees of obesity seem to be harmless. In the absence of other risk factors the weight must rise about 18 percent above the "normal" level before an insurance underwriter would begin to load the policy. Diabetes encourages the factors that generate atheroma, so there is every reason for being careful about its management.

Abnormally high blood pressure endangers life, particularly when it is associated with cigarette smoking, gross obesity, and high blood cholesterol and triglyceride levels; it is very reassuring to know that this cluster of risk factors is secondary to exhaustion and arousal in most cases, and can be reduced to an acceptable level or eradicated by measures that the individual can take.

Oral contraceptives are said to increase the risk of a coronary in women over the age of thirty-five, but it is not clear whether the risk applies to everyone or just to those who have already embarked on the downhill course towards a heart attack. It would seem a good precaution for "at risk" women, and certainly those who smoke, to change to another contraceptive method.

Exercise will be discussed under the heading of rehabilitation—but a person who keeps fit and tough enough to meet life's demands is more likely to keep healthy than the person who is exhausted repeatedly by the real and imaginary obligations accepted or undertaken.

The word "stress" has been used in a variety of ways by doctors. Some restrict it to psychological or social stimuli, rather than to physical factors such as heat and humidity. Many now use it to describe the feelings of discomfort or loss of self-esteem which are experienced when there is difficulty in keeping the actual performance up to its intended level.

The concept of "arousal" has the advantage of a simple English meaning (being stirred into activity) which fits the scientific meaning given to it by the researchers who study the responses of the brain and body to changing circumstances. Evidence is accumulating that atheroma and heart damage are closely related to an individual's response to life circumstances, and especially anything that threatens a loss of understanding and control of the environment, or a loss of command of personal "territory."

CORONARY BREAKDOWN—THE DANGER SIGNS

What then are the symptoms of exhaustion and ill health that precede a coronary breakdown? The signs may become recognizable six months, a year, or even more beforehand. Weariness is commonly generated by adverse changes at work and at home, changes that make existence an unusual struggle. Typically there are conflicts and alterations inflicted by others upon the customary way of life; actual or threatened loss of job; and bereavement. Moving the place of work takes its toll because it creates housing, commuting, and social problems. Being cut off from fellowship and kinship makes it harder to defend the health. Environmental factors such as heat waves and inflation increase the risk of heart attacks.

Of course, everyone facing adverse circumstances does not become ill. Patients who do have commonly made four mistakes. First, they have ignored the rule that neither military units nor people are designed to function indefinitely under unremitting and maximal effort: we all need to balance periods of intense effort with periods of low endeavor and slackness. Second, they have failed to organize an adequate amount of sleep. Third, they have failed to keep themselves fit and tough enough for their chosen lifestyles. Fourth, they have failed to realize that sheer willpower cannot overcome exhaustion and ill health—it can only act by increasing arousal, and producing a downward shift on the human function curve.

The reasons for a harmful level of overloading include an inability to say no to the demands of others, and a destructive level of greed for territory, power, or possessions. Exhausting overactivity may stem from insecurity and lack of self-esteem, or it may be a method of concealing an anxiety that is too threatening to be brought up into the conscious view.

Abnormal Tiredness

The earliest danger signs are subjective. The first group of symptoms are caused by the inability of the heart to produce the energy to meet all the demands of the active and aggressive individual. Principally there is an abnormal sort of tiredness which can overcome one's will and make it an increasing struggle to maintain the customary range of activities. Inessential pursuits have to be jettisoned. Abnormal sleeping habits develop, such as inability to keep awake during the evenings and to sleep properly through the night. This declining ability is either denied or attributed resentfully to the effects of aging.

One of the early South African heart transplant patients (Philip Blaiberg) described the symptoms well: "But in January 1967 the picture changed. I began to feel exhausted at my surgery. Work became a burden. With each passing day I needed more rest at home and between tending patients. I ascribed my state to overwork. Getting up in the mornings became increasingly difficult. I would walk to the station about ten minutes from my home . . . I now found even this short distance too much for me and so I used the car."

Shortly before his death, the author H. E. Bates was reported as saying: "I was so exhausted I thought I was going to have another coronary." Neither Bates nor Blaiberg spoke of pain when he gave his spontaneous accounts of growing disability. Most patients who undergo this sort of deterioration do not seek advice until their capacity for physical exercise has dropped to something less than twenty percent of its usual level. They do not seem to see it as a reparable fault and seek a cause, as they would if their motor cars developed a comparable drop in horsepower. The reason is probably the popular belief that nothing important can be going wrong in the absence of pain.

Unpleasant Sensations

The second group of symptoms also reflect the heart's waning ability to cope with physical and emotional challenges of life and are associated with its becoming swollen and distended when it is driven too hard. The swelling may not be sufficient to be seen on routine chest x-rays, but it is great enough to alter the heart pulsations and cause a steep rise in pressure within the wall of the left ventricular pump. It causes sensations that may be unpleasant or painful and difficult to ignore. The painful sensations are given the name *angina pectoris.*

Their best description was provided in *Circulation* in 1972 by Charles Friedberg:

> It is doubtful that the numerous descriptive terms indicating the quality of the pain are necessary for diagnosis, or indeed specific enough by themselves to be reliable. Neither is the exact location of the pain or its radiation absolutely essential for diagnosis. Major characteristics provide a minimal basis for accurate diagnosis.

> Pain, for which other terms such as pressure, tightness or heaviness may be substituted, or even breathlessness if this is associated with

any discomfort in the chest. Its location, though generally in the anterior or posterior chest, is less important provided it is not confined to the lower extremities or the head. Thus pain may represent *angina pectoris* even if it is confined to or located predominantly in the upper extremities or abdomen, provided that it is induced by walking rapidly or emotion. Radiation to the upper extremity or extremities, though helpful in excluding certain possible causes of chest pain, is not specific for *angina pectoris* since pain in the anterior chest and arm may be due to cervical radiculitis or to injury or strain of the pectoralis muscle. Radiation of chest pain to jaws, teeth or face provides some diagnostic specificity, but its sensitivity is low because of the relative infrequency of such radiation.

Precipitation of pain or pressure, etc., by walking outdoors (especially when hurrying, carrying a package or walking in cold weather or in a cold wind).

That a patient can walk or exercise indoors without pain, or that usually he can walk even long distances without discomfort, should not be interpreted to exclude *angina pectoris*. Not what the patient can usually do without the pain, but the circumstances at the moment when he does have pain are diagnostically decisive. If the pain occurs only occasionally, but specifically when walking to or from the subway, bus or car, and forces him to stop or slow down to obtain relief, then he has *angina pectoris,* whether or not he can walk a mile or more at other times. Often the patient walks so little or rarely that he is unaware of this relationship and he must be urged to use appropriate outdoor walking as a diagnostic test.

Precipitation of pain by emotion, especially when associated with acrimonious discussion or prolonged discussion on the telephone. The pain must develop in close time relationship to the precipitating emotional experience, not hours later.

Other Causes

Of course, fatigue and a fall in ability to cope with mental and physical challenges have many causes other than heart trouble. Depression is probably the most common cause of abnormal tiredness. Lack of training, cigarette smoking, chronic bronchitis, obesity, and anemia are probably the most frequent sources of a restricted capacity for physical effort.

Diagnosis

The diagnosis of heart trouble is a professional matter for a doctor, as is the choice of special tests that may be employed. Having the patient lie on his or her left side and then feeling and listening for signs of an abnormal heartbeat may be more useful than many highly technical tests. Some specialists record the heart pulsations and sounds in this position. The electrocardiogram, which traces the electrical activity of the heart, is universally employed, but some consider it less sensitive than the fingers and ears for detecting the early signs of coronary illness. It may remain normal during minor attacks of myocardial infarction or return quickly to normal afterwards. It can remain normal until after the onset of a major heart attack, and is therefore not a particularly good predictive test even when carried out after exercise. Coronary arteriography, that is the x-ray examination of the coronary arteries, is increasingly used as a diagnostic test, but the films do not tell us much about human function. For example, it is on record that one man with 99 percent, 95 percent and 80 percent narrowings of the three major coronary arteries reorganized his life and trained to become a marathon runner, whereas many others are locked into a state of painful disability even though the coronary narrowings might be no more than the average for urbanized middle-aged males.

WHAT TO DO

A glance at the human function curve makes it obvious that the only way out of ill health or breakdown caused by excessive and prolonged arousal and unrelieved exhaustion is to reduce the arousal to an acceptable level and to remove the exhaustion.

Today's urban warriors react against the obvious because they are bent only on their attempt to close the gap between the actual performance and their intentions. Instead of standing back and taking stock of their resources and circumstances they usually demand the removal of symptoms and readily take drugs to lower the blood pressure, and to remove the pain of angina. Sometimes they even demand coronary artery bypass grafting (a surgical treatment in which pieces of vein are employed to bypass coronary arterial narrowings) to remove pain, hoping perhaps that the operation's bypassing of some of the debris of the past can provide them with immunity against the effects of their using themselves destructively in the future.

For this reason it is worthwhile to show the warrior and his (or her) spouse a gymnasium where former patients are training to lose their disability and to become capable of much more healthy activity than they could achieve in the year or so before the threat of *angina pectoris* or myocardial infarction entered their lives. The visit to the gymnasium usually satisfies the warrior that the illness is not the beginning of a cabbage-like existence, but rather nature's call for the reorganization of life into a happier and more efficient mode. Once the anxiety and exhaustion have been dealt with it is amazing how often the real and imaginary obstacles to the reorganization shrink down to a manageable size and open the way to a more successful life.

Facing the Facts

At some stage the warriors must open their eyes to the fact that going out of action temporarily to rest and retrain is a very different matter from struggling on in a sick way and using drugs to remove symptoms: they are always entitled to ask whether the purpose of any proposed treatment is to strengthen their coping ability or to remove the warnings of a destructive lifestyle. Unfortunately for the doctor's peace of mind, most warriors resist change because their pride in past achievement inclines them to deny the need for change. They want to hold on to every tactic that has helped them to reach their station in life, irrespective of whether it has led to premature bankruptcy of health.

The reduction of arousal and the removal of exhaustion may take the form of an urgent rescue operation or a longer-term management program according to the individual's proximity to a breakdown. The quickest way of reducing arousal in an emergency is to put the patient into a comfortable sleep with an intravenous injection; this can be lifesaving in acute coronary insufficiency or myocardial infarction where the rapidly escalating demands of anxiety and pain are outstripping the pumping ability of the heart and causing deterioration from pain, lung congestion, irregular heart action, or incipient failure of the circulation. The second quickest way of reducing arousal is for an able doctor to take command of the circumstances and produce order out of disarray.

In less urgent rescue operations the agitated arousal that threatens the heart can yield to reassurance and support. "Recharging the batteries" with rich and generous sleep can bring about a quick recovery from a temporary swing towards a coronary breakdown. For example, one hard-working middle-aged man became ill with heart pain when his son-in-law threatened to take his business from him. His heart became distended, and his blood pressure and serum cholesterol rose alarmingly. It looked as though he was well on the way into his second myocardial infarction. On March 18 measures were taken to provide good old-fashioned nursing care combined with an excellent quality of sleeping from one mealtime to the next. By March 22 the pain had gone, the heart had lost its over-distention, the blood pressure had fallen to its usual level, the cholesterol had come down, and he was able to face his problems with calm determination.

These sorts of swings towards a coronary breakdown are rarely spontaneous. The difficulty in finding and dealing with the cause lies in the human tendency to deny its existence, and sometimes years may pass before one learns whom the patient blamed for the breakdown. Nevertheless, the swing is much more often attributable to a failure to act intelligently in difficult circumstances than it is to cardiac damage coming out of the blue.

Supportive Convalescence

If the patient has no natural support group in his corner, perhaps because he has isolated himself from loving relationships, or has suffered bereavement, it is necessary to create one from voluntary or professional resources. It is increasingly difficult these days to achieve the conditions required for the wounds of urban society to heal in peace, and the attempt commonly demands more of the cardiologist's time and skill than the prescription of drugs. The task was easier when nurses trained in the Florence Nightingale tradition knew how to preserve and increase a patient's delicate resources; when hospitals were smaller and less expensive to run; and when communities accepted the need to look after the sick at home.

Taking Stock

After the rescue operation has been carried out in the hospital or the home, and the anxiety has been looked after, it is necessary to take stock of the factors which brought on the attack. There is little point in someone crawling off prematurely to fight the same old battle with the same old tactics that had been tried and proved inadequate. To quote Sir James Mackenzie again: "Treatment for *angina pectoris* requires careful enquiry into the conditions including exhaustion. First and foremost a stop must be put to that form of exertion which has induced the attack, and any other conditions that predispose to it must be avoided, such as worry, sleeplessness, overindulgence in food and alcohol, tobacco. . . . Attacks of *angina pectoris* may be directly induced by want of refreshing sleep, and may be stopped by measures taken to induce sleep . . . IT MAY BE TAKEN AS AN AXIOM THAT IF THE PATIENT DOES NOT GET SUFFICIENT SLEEP, HE WILL NEVER GET WELL." I do not believe that the passage of time has made these observations any less valid.

Taking stock of the behavior and the circumstances that brought about the defeat is helped by talking to a sympathetic and intelligent but not sycophantic listener. The process stirs up the emotions and may cause an outbreak of weeping. This is not weakness, but a very good start to the recovery. It is useful to read one patient's words:

> The heart attack did not come out of the blue, as these attacks are supposed to do: the ground was prepared by faulty living and the attack itself was in a way self-induced. This is not mere fancy—it is the result of much reading, enquiry, self-examination and analysis, and careful deduction from known facts. I know for a certainty that I shall never have another heart attack unless in some way it is brought about by me, either by allowing my physical condition to degenerate, my mind and body to become overtired and overtaxed, or by permitting a too personal and subjective reaction to some situation of stress. This conviction has relieved my mind of its most potent weapon for destruction: worry . . .

> Stage two on my road back to health was the ability at last to learn to "box clever"—that is, to deal with all stressful situations, whatever their nature, intelligently and constructively, or else calmly to refuse to have anything to do with them. This implies a degree of mental awareness and self-control which is difficult to cultivate but which, with perseverance, will always come. Instead of reacting to a situation with emotion—one reacts with reason. In matters involving personalities one comes to understand other people better, to see more of them, as it were. Situations which contain the seeds of hostility undergo a subtle and significant change: in fact, life itself takes on altogether more significance.

> (From *Coronary Case* by R. Edwards, Faber & Faber 1964.)

In the early stage of recovery the coronary patient who is learning to keep arousal down to the level that will permit recovery may complain of frustration because he or she cannot do enough to allay guilt and anxiety or to provide security. There is no point in allowing the arousal from this source to carry the patient over into exhaustion and ill health all over again—it should be brought home that this period of resting allows the heart to grow a rich network of bypass arteries, and accepting this is the first step in the process of training.

It is very uncommon for spontaneous outcrops of heart damage to hold up progress at this stage. Almost always a setback is self-induced by an uncalculated outburst of physical or emotional effort. At the other extreme are those who never make the most of themselves after coronary illness because they cannot be liberated from the family anxiety. A well-supervised program of rehabilitation is the common sense answer to the problem of finding the best practical course of activity.

HOW TO MINIMIZE THE RISK OF A CORONARY

The essence of keeping well and avoiding a coronary breakdown is for each individual to learn to use his healthy function to a maximum, not fearing the initiative, persistence, leadership and hard work that are required for success and not fearing healthy tiredness; but using vigilance, self-awareness and skill to avoid self-defeating excesses of arousal and exhaustion. It is axiomatic that the body must be kept fit enough and tough enough for the demands of the mind.

Some humans have a greater taste for self-defeating excesses of arousal and exhaustion than others. A "coronary" behavior pattern may be extremely rewarding from a materialistic point of view, but it offers the individual little happiness and solves few problems in a satisfactory manner. This person is constantly drawn into new situations in which he or she creates competition. These sorts of people have been called workaholics, and Aldous Huxley described them as adrenalin-addicted. Addiction to work and tension is the chief impediment to cardiac rehabilitation.

It is particularly necessary for those with this type of personality to guard against exhaustion, because self-awareness and self-control slip away very quickly under the effects of high arousal and sleep deprivation.

Working Environment

Coronary heart disease seems to occur with greater frequency in individuals who tend to work harder and longer hours than others. The proportion of time during which a coronary-prone person works compared with the time during which he relaxes, sleeps, eats, or pursues hobbies, is higher than with other individuals, and the amount of work performed is often greater than that done by others. Work seems to be deeply involved in the patient's sense of duty and conscience. Very striking is the tendency to accept challenges and so to assume more tasks than can leisurely be fulfilled; to accept, for example, a tight deadline and then feel obliged to keep the promise. Such people sacrifice leisure and family life to fulfill an almost compulsive urge to work more and more. Work seems to be the main way in which they strive to climb the social scale. Many of them have achieved higher social positions than their parents (who gave them an example of dutifulness); they attribute this to their hard and conscientious work.

They also demonstrate another characteristic behavior pattern—a tendency to dominate others. They strive towards or fight for power and leadership. The tendency to assume responsibility can also be seen as an expression of this striving to dominate. Especially during middle age they, more than others, channel their aggression into hard work.

Family Environment

The same striving for power is seen in the family setting—sometimes interpreted by the individual concerned as a sense of responsible leadership. He expects wife and children to submit to him, to respect him, and to give him the love to which he is entitled as a recompense for his hard work and care. Actually, underlying the tendency towards "partriarchal domination," there is a great need for love from wife and children, but this is rarely admitted.

Community Participation

These coronary-prone individuals are found more often in occupations in which climbing the social ladder can result from hard responsible work. They seem to take a more active part in the social life of the community, smoke more cigarettes, drive bigger cars, be more "involved." Many are driven to these communal activities by the same conscience and responsibility that drives them into hard work for their families. In their hobbies, which are seldom relaxing, the same hyperactivity is evident. Some do intensive sports to show that they can still teach younger people a lesson. Also, in their sexual life they have to prove to themselves and others that they are active and vigorous—by doing so they often ask too much from themselves. They do not like to appeal to others for help in difficult situations and often believe that in modern society every person has to fight for a position. They maintain less warm contacts with their extended family, so that in difficult times they receive less support than others from relatives and friends. They tend to fight financial difficulties—like other challenges—on their own as long as possible and often keep worries to themselves. On the whole they strive for "male" achievements; their ideal is to be strong, admired, and invulnerable; their fear is to appear fearful, weak, old, dependent, and "feminine." Passive wishes are unacceptable and therefore repressed, but are voiced to a doctor when they are given an opportunity to unburden. Actually these persons are greatly in need of love and much of their striving is devoted to obtaining power as a substitute for love. As one of them put it: "I am a big fellow with a small heart."

Interhuman Conflicts

The heart attack often seems to occur after an emotional conflict; sometimes acute and severe, but in many cases only one of a series of apparently trivial irritations. The essence of this conflict is a frustration of the tendency to dominate at work or in the family, or both, coupled with frustration of the desire for admiration and social recognition. There may have been a failure (real or threatening) to ascent of the social ladder; a setback in salary or position at work; disobedience or lack of submission by wife or children; chronic or recurrent financial worries or a real or threatening acute financial catastrophe— all this occurring in spite of hard and intensive work which in the view of the subjects should have called for recompense rather than for frustration. Most people of this temperament react to the frustration, as to every challenge, by working even harder. They sometimes express this as fighting back after being driven to the wall, the frustration seeming to be worse if it is the very person whom the individual expected to submit to him, or to appreciate him, who puts him in a position in which he has to submit himself—for example, a wife who refused intercourse or who dominated, criticized, interrupted, or "corrected" the husband in the presence of others; a too-independent son or daughter; a domineering business partner or boss; a rival who wins out by unfair competition. (See *Modern Trends in Psychosomatic Medicine* by J. J. Groen, London 1976).

High Score You Lose

The life change scoring techniques came into being in 1967 when T. H. Holmes and R. H. Rahe (see *Journal of Psycho-*

somatic Medicine) concluded that people make valid judgments about the amount and duration of changes in the accustomed pattern of life produced by the events taking place around them. Giving an arbitrary 50 points to marriage, Holmes and Rahe found it possible to make a scale of events that disturbed the customary patterns of life. (The scale is shown on pages 85 and 86.)

It is not possible to quote any particular score as a danger level because individuals vary so much in their capacity to withstand breakdown from large and persistent life change scores, and because each individual's resistance diminishes as the position on the personal function curve shifts downward towards the point of breakdown. Nevertheless, a half-yearly score of about sixty units and a yearly score of more than 150 might be regarded as inviting ill health. It is commonplace to find that patients approaching a coronary breakdown have been exhausted by the struggle against scores on the order of 400 to 600 for two or three years.

POINTS

100	death of a spouse
73	divorce
60–69	marital separation, imprisonment, death of a close relative
50–59	personal injury or illness
50	marriage
40–49	loss of job, marital reconciliation, retirement, change in health of a family member, pregnancy
30–39	sex difficulties, new family member, business readjustment, change in financial condition, death of close friend, change to a different line of work, change in number of arguments with spouse, large mortgage
20–29	foreclosure of mortgage or loan, change in responsibilities at work, son or daughter leaving home, trouble with in-laws, out-

standing personal achievement, wife begins or stops work, change in living conditions, revision of personal habits, trouble with boss, change in work hours or conditions, change in residence

10-19   changes in recreation, church or school activities, small mortgage, minor violation of law, change in eating/sleeping habits, and number of family get-togethers, vacation, Christmas.

Environmental Factors

Environmental pollution can be another major cause of the excessive arousal that leads to exhaustion, ill health, and coronary breakdown. The death rate is increased with measurable changes such as heat waves and economic crises, and the level of arousal can be raised by unpleasant noise, but the pollutants we are most closely concerned with cannot be measured. The most important seem to be the challenges and threats against the individual achieving and maintaining the mastery of his circumstances and territory. Common examples are people-poisoning (recurrent unpleasant tension induced by people from whom escape is not possible); affliction with difficult time pressures; and resentment about changes made against one's will by others in families, communities, and hierarchical organizations.

Overcrowding is an important cause of arousal in urban life. The unpleasant tension in, say, a crowded underground train depends not only upon the number of people in the carriage and the rate of changing at stations, but also upon the amount of space and privacy required by each individual for peace of mind, and the nature of the other passengers.

Mental Overload

Another common cause of excessive arousal, ill health and breakdown is "information input overloading," that is, an overloading of the brain with messages that require attention and action (or withholding from action). The ability of the brain to cope with the message is limited by its circuitry and is affected by the individual's position on a personal human function curve. There are several reasons for persistent overloading. Some are unavoidable, as when a crisis produces too much information or information that is too novel or complex. But most of the persistent overloading related to coronary breakdown is controllable by the individual. One person may lack judgment and generate more action than can be controlled. A second may feel insecure and be unable to refuse the overwhelming demands of others because of the need for their approval. A third may outstrip health reserves in an impatient desire to achieve too much too soon.

Konrad Lorenz has studied the environmental factors responsible for increasing the level of aggression in everyday life. His list includes overcrowding; violence; commercial competitiveness and status seeking; militant enthusiasm and righteousness (for which political parties exist); rapid ecological and social changes making the traditional approaches to problems useless and rendering the elders unfit to lead; and a breakdown of morality from hunger, anxiety, endlessly facing difficult decisions, overwork, and helplessness. These sources of arousal, creating ill health and breakdown, are much more likely to be the cause of the upsurge of coronary disease in areas of rapid urbanization and westernization than a change in eating habits.

Avoidance and Survival Tactics

It is easier to do well and to survive the common dangers when the qualities required for success are abundant, and this requires the individual to organize himself and his circumstances in such a way as to stay in the healthy part of the human function curve. It usually means that one has to remain the master and not the slave of circumstances. The techniques can be examined in sequence.

The first is the ability to make an audit or appraisal of one's real standing, relationships, and resources. It may not be so important to achieve accurate self-knowledge when the reserves of strength and energy seem to be infinite, but there is no place for self-deception when it is necessary to avoid or to recover from a breakdown.

If the audit reveals a position on the downward slope of the human function curve it is essential to acquire the discipline to reduce arousal and remove exhaustion. Without this discipline everything is left to chance. Everyone must find ways for dealing with overloading, people-poisoning, and pressures of time in order to make life comfortable enough for survival. Most people find it much easier to struggle on until they drop than to withdraw from battle at times of their own choosing. Guilt often makes them feel that their failure to meet their targets must be punished by harder striving or painful operations: they do not see that more can be achieved in the long run if they withdraw to relax and rest back into healthy function when exhaustion is making them ill and inefficient.

An essential part of the discipline is the ability to foresee and to rearrange events that might cause too steep a rise in the life change score. For example, retiring from work and moving immediately to a new house in a strange district might cause a breakdown that could be avoided by delaying the move for some months. If the events cannot be rearranged it is usually possible to build up reserves of energy beforehand, providing the will and the understanding exist.

Sleep Is Essential

Discipline is also required to produce good sleep in hard times. Whatever form the heart failure may assume, sleep is essential: "It may be taken as an axiom that if the patient does not get sufficient sleep he will never get well." Good sleep is the best first-line defense for the coronary-prone individual threatened with ill health or breakdown. Sleeping soundly for a few nights, and perhaps through a Sunday morning and afternoon can make a wonderful difference to the individual who is slipping downwards into ill health. Two or three 5 mg Valium tablets taken for sleeping at times of need appears to be safe, effective, and nonaddictive. In extremely threatening circumstances this dose may be inadequate, but higher doses must not be taken except on medical advice. A sense of languor the next day is not a contraindication because it helps to achieve restfulness until the "batteries are charged."

Self-help

One of the best ways of achieving a greater workload without succumbing to arousal and exhaustion is to become fitter and tougher, and consequently capable of greater energy output.

When unacceptable resentment, frustration, and loss of command dominate life it is common for a diagnosis of depression to be made. However, this state of unbearable frustration is not melancholia, and antidepressant medicines are not the answer. It is better to deal effectively with the sleep deprivation and allow the patient's support group to talk him or her through the bad time. Sometimes a professional can bring peace of mind in unbearable circumstances, and instruction in the technique of relaxation (that is, reducing arousal) has saved many of my patients from burning themselves down into another breakdown.

Friedman has advised the coronary type of men and women to stop doing more than one thing at a time; to learn to listen without interrupting; to escape into books that demand concentration; to learn to eat slowly and savor the food; to have a private retreat in the home; to plan some idleness every day; to eradicate people-poisoning wherever possible; and to organize business trips and vacations in such a way as to avoid time pressures.

AFTER A CORONARY

To rehabilitate is to "set up again in proper conditions," and no words could express more clearly the need of a person who has approached or suffered a coronary breakdown. To be set up again in healthy conditions implies that healthy human function can be achieved and maintained if the individual respects the inexorable laws of nature and chooses not to force himself into the over-aroused and exhausted lifestyle which generates self-defeating changes in the blood and blood pressure.

In the 1960s an interested observer could see enormous individual variations in the recovery from coronary breakdown: some were failures because fear and family pressures made them adventure too little, others because a variant of the same fear drove them into wild excesses of uncontrolled arousal. A few were outstanding successes and ten years later seemed to be healthier and happier, physically more active, and more efficient in the business of living and making a living than they ever were before the illness was diagnosed. These successful patients had little regard for the pharmacological fashion of the day. Their results seemed not to be related to the severity or duration of the breakdown, but to depend upon the intuitive way in which their life had been reorganized. Their principles were to make an objective audit of their behavior and circumstances, to disconnect health from sources of excessive arousal, and to train methodically to become fit enough for the success that they needed.

It seemed reasonable to create a training program for persons who wished to benefit from these principles, and Alistair Murray, director of the City Gym Research Unit in London, proved an efficient trainer. In the 1960s it seemed strange to some authorities that training in a particular gymnasium should be prescribed for coronary patients, but it was obvious that the optimum level of physical activity could be achieved more efficiently by training under supervision than by untutored adventures in the local park. Some objected that the study of heart function in relation to human function would generate cardiac neurosis among coronary patients, but one knew that trainee military parachutists, similarly going forward into the unknown, derived great comfort from the motto "Knowledge Dispels Fear."

Preparation for Rehabilitation

Before patients are accepted for training in a rehabilitation gymnasium they should be observed over a two-month testing period of pre-treatment, during which they learn to obtain adequate sleep, to live without exhaustion, and to avoid excessive arousal. They also learn to avoid the physical and emotional circumstances that produce heart pain. As they learn to avoid angina and cardiac discomfort they learn to do without their drug treatment. Anyone expressing dependence upon these tablets is startled by the improvement that comes from controlling arousal, obtaining adequate sleep, and refusing to produce angina. A tenfold gain in walking ability within three or four weeks is a commonplace event. They are not nagged to lose weight or to stop smoking in this period because the reorganization of their life and attitudes provides a large enough challenge to their coping ability. Professional tuition in relaxation is available for those who are unable to achieve it on their own.

A person who passes the pre-treatment phase successfully, learns to live comfortably without drugs and chooses to attend for training, meets three influences at the gymnasium. One is the teaching about the effects of arousal and exhaustion upon performance. The second is the informal discussion over refreshments where new members can learn tactics for avoiding exhaustion from those who have been successful. It is by no means assumed that the world is going to get better for anyone: all must learn to make successful use of their own coping ability. The third influence is the exercise itself.

The heart rate is taken before activity at the gymnasium and no work is done until it has relaxed down to less than 90 beats a minute. The first work is a test dose of light mobilizing exercises calculated not to put the heart rate above 100/min. The patient is closely watched for any hint of discomfort or strain. The response to the test enables the trainer to judge whether the person is ready for exercise training and to choose a program that fits age and observed condition.

The exercise program commonly consists of a series of ten rhythmical and submaximal movements carried out for fifteen to twenty minutes, three times a week for two months. The loads employed and the speed, variety, and number of movements are calculated to keep the heart rate within prescribed limits. The schedules permit a progressive increase in comfortable activity which can be continued until the patient reaches an optimal level. Competition between members does not take place because each is concentrating solely upon personal achievements. The general atmosphere is warm and comfortable and dispels the notion that spartan conditions are required for physical training.

The first result of the training is a change of attitude. The patient becomes more relaxed and confident as he or she sees a positive way back into healthy function, loses the conviction that previous disability was an irremovable mark of aging, and loses a sense of guilt about neglecting health.

Sooner or later in the course of training almost everyone forgets to organize sleeping time and allows arousal or overwork to exhaust him. This is one of the most valuable lessons because it shows what a large effect such lack of discipline can have upon the level of fitness that has been achieved, and teaches the individual when to choose to rest instead of exercising. Through the training the patient learns to translate gymnasium activity to the world outside and thereby to judge the desirable amount of walking, stair-climbing, gardening, and so forth. One also learns to recognize when one is ready for work and to gauge how much can be done without the risk of deterioration. The signs of successful rehabilitation are obvious. They include a relaxed manner, enjoyment of physical exercise, and loss of the old guilt-reaction to the idea of investing time in relaxation and exercise.

DISORDERS OF THE HEART RATE AND RHYTHM

The conscious mind is not usually aware of the heartbeat unless severe exertion, excitement, or the changes produced by a hot bath or altitude, for example, make it pound strongly, and this rarely causes alarm because the sensations are perceived as a reasonable response to the circumstances.

However, it is quite easy for a healthy person to become "tuned in" to the heartbeat in such a way as to be keenly aware of fluctuations in the rate and the extra beats which are a part of normal life. This hypersensitive awareness tends to come during periods of exhaustion and mental overloading when the force of the heartbeat and the tendency to extra beats may be heightened. Under these conditions the patient becomes convinced that an abnormal heartbeat is the *cause* not the *symptom* of an ill-fitting life: it can be very difficult to persuade the sufferer that the symptoms do not indicate heart disease. The best course is to deal with the arousal, remove the exhaustion and sleep deprivation, and provide a course of physical training that will recover fitness and restore confidence.

Paroxysmal tachycardia is the name given to bursts of rapid beating which result from runs of extra beats going on for minutes, hours or days, and these are more commonly derived from severe degrees of exhaustion and arousal than from heart disease.

Rapid regular or irregular beating that presents a persistent or recurring problem or causes disability should be investigated. The physician may find a toxic condition such as thyroid overactivity or alcoholism, for example, or an established heart disorder such as atrial fibrillation. When the doctor has provided the appropriate treatment, the patient should learn how to make the best of himself. The first step is to recognize the degree of arousal and exhaustion that invites attacks, and the second is to reorganize life style in order to avoid it. The best preventive measure is to sleep well, and the best treatment for an actual attack is to get rid of anxious associations and to go off into a satisfying sleep with the help of a sleeping pill or tranquilizer if the doctor thinks it advisable.

Excessive slowing of the heart rate causes an inadequate amount of blood to be pumped to the brain. Confusion and loss of consciousness are the common consequences that may be seen in partial or complete fainting attacks. These fainting attacks are responses: exhaustion and anxiety may play a part in predisposing some individuals to fainting, while others are sensitive to the sight of blood or scenes of horror. Associated with the slowing may be an excessive pooling of blood in the legs, as in the case of the man getting out of a warm bed quickly to stand and urinate, or a soldier collapsing on the parade ground.

The best first-aid treatment is to lay the individual on the floor on the back and raise the legs to encourage blood to flow back to the heart. The head should be turned to one side to ensure that stomach contents will be spilled out and not inhaled into the lungs if vomiting takes place. False teeth should be removed and the breathing passages cleared of any obstruction. If the pulse does not return immediately the breast bone should be given two or three slaps with the flat of the hand. If the pulse still does not return the treatment should be given as for cardiac arrest, namely closed-chest massage and mouth-to-mouth inflation of the lungs.

If an intrinsic defect of the heart's pacemaking and rate-controlling equipment is responsible for losses of consciousness, it is logical and practical to provide treatment by an operation to insert an electrical pacemaker.

LOW BLOOD PRESSURE

It is not intended to discuss here the low blood pressure that forms part of acute emergencies such as hemorrhage, crush injury, cholera, and myocardial infarction, but to comment on the "low blood pressure" which is offered as an explanation for symptoms of debility. In the United Kingdom and the United States this is more commonly regarded as a matter for congratulation because actuaries view low blood pressure favorably. The only symptom the executive is likely to encounter is giddiness or faintness on coming upright from a sitting or lying position. If the symptom is severe or persistent a medical search is needed for the rare conditions which prevent normal blood pressure adjusting to changes of posture. When these have been excluded the problem can usually be solved by adding more table salt to the diet and getting up slowly after a few moments of leg-bracing exercises.

NORMAL AND HIGH BLOOD PRESSURE

Blood pressure is the term used to describe the pressure within the arterial tubes. It rises and falls with each heartbeat; the sphygmomanometer applied to the arm is the usual method for recording the higher (systolic) and lower (diastolic) level in millimeters of mercury. A host of factors related to arousal, physical activity, and the stiffness of the arteries can change the systolic and diastolic levels. Few people in a crowd will have identical blood pressures because the differences between individuals and the fluctuations within any one individual are very great. In some the rises last for minutes and may be caused by anxiety about the medical examination. In others the rises can last for months or years in relation to their behavior and circumstances.

There is no sharp dividing line between normal and abnormally high blood pressure (hypertension). Life insurance companies tend to use a level of 140/90 even though this level may be found among half the men over fifty years of age. A recent survey of Swedish males aged forty-seven to fifty-four years showed that 16 percent had hypertension severe enough to reduce their life expectancy by eleven years in actuarial terms. About 5 percent of tenth-grade students in Chicago had systolic pressures of 150 or more or diastolic levels of 90 or more.

There is good reason to follow the principle that the blood pressure will tend to stay up when it is worked up often. The more often it is given a chance to relax down the more difficult it will be for circumstances to put it up again.

In spite of massive research little has been learned in this century about the causes of high blood pressure, probably because it has been fashionable to study the inner workings of the body without looking deeply into the effects of behavior and circumstances. In 1909 T. Lauder Brunton, who understood the effects of adrenalin on the circulation, pointed out that hurry and worry, and above all angry emotion, raised the blood pressure very greatly. After a lifetime of research Sir George Pickering summed up the position by saying:

> We are beginning to learn that certain situations in life elevate the arterial pressure . . . it is likely that at least some of them will be definable in terms of the behavior of the mind. The more frequent these situations, and the longer they last, the higher will be the arterial pressure.

Kidney disease and other "organic" causes of hypertension probably account for 5 percent of the problem in executives. In another 5 percent the blood pressure probably remains up because permanent changes have set in due to its being worked up for long periods over many years. In the remainder no "organic disease" changes are found and the blood pressure can settle down to a normal level with the removal of exhaustion and the management of arousal, that is, when conditions of mental and physical rest are achieved. A week of resting in a warm and caring atmosphere with sleep induced in the mornings, the afternoons and at night is a good test. In well over half the cases the resting and relaxation produce long-lasting changes, and the blood pressure remains down when the patient goes forward in an intelligently planned and easier way. Rehabilitation helps to expand the ability to work without regenerating exhaustion and hypertension.

In the others something more must be done if the patient is not simply to return with unchanged attitudes to the same exhausting and provocative circumstances. Therapy is difficult. Drugs are usually disliked on principle, and in any case do not help all patients. The chief problem is that a dose suitable for low arousal days is not strong enough to be effective on high arousal days, and a dose that controls the blood pressure on high arousal days produces unacceptable side effects on the others.

Once it has been demonstrated that the hypertension is not organically based, and will yield to the management of arousal and exhaustion, it is reasonable to give the patient the responsibility for managing the condition. The patient can be taught how to deal with arousal and to overcome sleep deprivation, and can be given thiazide diuretics to reduce the amount of salt in the body; but only he or she can make the day-to-day choices of action that determine whether he or she remains in the healthy part of the function curve and enjoys normal blood pressure, or goes over into exhaustion, ill health, and hypertension. There is little difficulty in teaching a willing executive to record his or her blood pressure. There is great therapeutic pleasure in seeing an intelligent person learn to work and fight successfully without putting blood pressure up to actuarially unacceptable levels; and little pleasure in trying to find a combination of pills that satisfy someone who is "killing" himself and making the lives of those around him a misery. There will be an important place in medicine for the counseling techniques that teach people to work efficiently without screwing themselves into habits that shorten their lives.

Throughout the world extensive trials are being made of beta-blocking drugs for hypertension and angina, and coronary artery bypass grafting operations for painful heart disability, and it will take some years to establish their rightful place. Basic principles and common sense suggest that these powerful interventions can be used as supplements in certain cases, but never as substitutes for the measures described here.

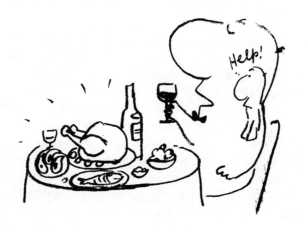

chapter 6

THE INNER PERSON

The belly is not only the site of much disease but a sounding-board to the emotions. Indeed, symptoms due to stress are nearly as common as those due to disease. Moreover, many people are more aware of their guts than of any other part of their body—partly because these upsets are so common that we all experience them at some time or other: indigestion, wind, heartburn, nausea, vomiting, constipation, or diarrhea.

Misunderstandings about the digestive system and how it works are surpisingly widespread. Many people have wrong ideas about the tongue, food, acid, bile, the liver, bowel, and so on. Understanding the facts should relieve anxiety.

Research in this field is active and is opening the door to better treatment. Hitherto, doctors have had to give advice based on tradition, but today advice can more often be guided by the findings of controlled research trials, and doctors can avoid interfering with the patient's way of life unnecessarily. In the past the treatment was sometimes worse than the complaint!

Many symptoms are due to stress, but the importance of this in causing duodenal ulcer, for example, has been exaggerated. Indeed, businesspeople, however much worry they have, can be reassured that they are no more prone to develop these disorders than anyone else. We know now that some troubles in the gut are really diseases of "civilized" societies caused by the type of food we eat.

STRESS AND THE GUT

Nerves and tension can cause symptoms such as indigestion and diarrhea. Also, as the mind can alter the working of the gut, worry probably makes ulcers worse. These psychosomatic disorders often occur in the best people: perfectionists in responsible positions who are conscientious and capable. They may have other nervous symptoms: fatigue, irritability, headaches, loss of interest in sex, and sleeplessness.

Patients may be advised to avoid worry and stress. However, to be effective this advice ought to be accompanied by the gift of a suitable income, a carefree job, and perhaps even the provision of a different spouse! Some, however, are able to take a more philosophical attitude and modify their reactions to the usual inevitable stresses of life. A variety of interests and hobbies creates a more tranquil mind than is usually possible when a person is obsessively devoted to work alone.

THE ROLE OF DIETS

It is not surprising that a link has been assumed between food and stomach trouble. This may indeed occur with certain foods that, handled without proper care and hygiene, convey germs, but with one or two exceptions food does not in itself cause disease. In the past, many patients have been quite unnecessarily deprived of the enjoyment of eating in fruitless attempts by doctors to help or cure them.

Research carefully carried out in the United Kingdom has shown that patients suffering from a peptic ulcer who dieted strictly did no better than those who ate and drank normally. There is also no reason why those with gall-bladder trouble should not be allowed to eat fat unless they are overweight or it upsets them, which is unusual. In the past, a low residue diet has been prescribed for those with large bowel (colon) disorders such as irritable colon or diverticulitis (which causes pain and bowel upsets). It was thought that small seeds and skins caused irritation and made pain or diarrhea worse. Studies now show that the opposite is the fact: that this part of the gut especially needs bulk and additional roughage to make it function properly.

The diet we choose can be an important cause of disease of the colon such as irritable colon, diverticulosis and -itis, and even perhaps cancer—as well as being responsible for constipation and piles (hemorrhoids). Evidence for this comes from a study of the geographical distribution of these diseases. The prime cause is the lack of fiber in the refined Western diet; for example, diverticulosis is hardly ever seen in under-developed countries, where plenty of vegetables and fruit are eaten instead of refined carbohydrates, sugar, white flour, and confectionery. Unknown in rural African communities, it develops in Africans when they live in towns. Moreover, blacks who eat the same food as other inhabitants of the United States developed diverticulosis like the rest. When fed on a refined diet rats also develop diverticulosis. The purpose of the large bowel is to retain waste matter, and when bulk is lacking the muscle contracts and tightens, producing balloon-like bulges at weak points (as in damaged bicycle tires) called diverticula. When bulk is added to the diet, the muscle of the large bowel relaxes and works properly.

The easiest way of adding bulk to food is by bran, the outer coating of wheat germ, which is removed when white flour is made. It is best when the fiber is coarsely ground as in miller's bran (unprocessed bran). Those suffering from constipation, irritable colon, and diverticulosis should therefore add bran to their food, and there is a case for all in the western-ized world being encouraged to eat more fiber (roughage). Bran itself can be bought from health stores and some grocers and supermarkets, and is pleasant with milk (adding raisins or nuts if wished), water, or fruit juice. Bran goes well with commer-cially available muesli, mixed half and half. It can be added to cereals, porridge, or soup. In making bread, twenty-five percent bran can be added to the wholemeal flour. Some (a dessertspoon or more) can be eaten with each meal. Fiber is also added by eating porridge or bran cereal, the stone ground instead of white loaf, green vegetables, and especially cabbage, root vegetables (potatoes should be eaten in their jackets) and salads—as well as fresh and dried fruit. The average portion of vegetables should be doubled or trebled.

EATING FOR PLEASURE

Appetite is a pleasant feeling linked with the thought of food, whereas hunger is disagreeable and associated with hunger-pangs, sometimes caused by an empty stomach contracting. Appetite does not always mean that the body needs food: the food eaten depends on social habits, and people usually eat more than they need; hence obesity is an almost exclusively human disease.

Appetite is increased by seeing and smelling food, by fresh air, exercise, and aperitifs such as sherry—also by an overactive thyroid gland, as in thyrotoxicosis. A person who suddenly starts eating enormous quantities may be suffering from a nervous disorder.

Loss of appetite is usual in diseases causing fever, anemia, and weakness. But loss of appetite with fastidiousness about food is often part of the make-up of neurotic patients. An extreme example of this is called *anorexia nervosa*; although it especially afflicts young women with emotional upsets, the disease seems to be affecting men with emotional problems too. Loss of appetite is also common in depression.

TEETH AND THEIR FUNCTION

Teeth are needed because food should be chewed properly before being swallowed. The large back teeth, the molars, grind food after it has been chopped up by the sharp incisors at the front. Good teeth are needed for good looks and in maintaining morale as well as for chewing.

Decay (dental caries) is very common, but as no one knows a cure, prevention is all important. Ancient and primitive races have been free from dental decay because they chew so much and their food contains little sugar.

In so-called civilized societies foods are more refined and contain little residue. Chewing cleans the teeth, and soft foods are swallowed without chewing. Another cause of dental decay is that bits of sugar and confectionery tend to lodge between the teeth, especially if the teeth are not brushed regularly, and provide food needed for the growth of germs (bacteria) which produce acid that attacks the enamel on teeth. Using a toothpick or dental floss may be advisable for cleaning any spaces between the teeth.

Teeth should be cleaned at least twice daily, using a toothbrush with up and down strokes (away from the gums), and no food should be eaten after brushing them at night. The most promising public health measure for preventing dental decay is for a trace of fluoride to be added to drinking water. Fluoridation is harmless and prevents dental decay. Nowadays, dental surgeons try to preserve teeth whenever possible, so regular visits are important. When dentures do become necessary they must fit well, otherwise it is not unknown for the patient to wear them for social reasons but take them out to eat.

Septic teeth are unpleasant but do not make people feel unwell, cause indigestion, rheumatism, or any other disease. In the past, extraction of teeth was advised for treating some diseases because bad teeth were thought to be the cause. This idea has been shown to be wrong. But special care is required for those whose heart valves have been affected by rheumatic fever; when teeth are extracted these people require penicillin or another antibiotic just before the extraction, to deal with the germs (otherwise harmless inhabitants of the gums) that are let loose in the blood. This does not matter in a healthy person, but if a heart valve is damaged germs may lodge on it and cause a serious and prolonged illness.

WHY SALIVA IS NEEDED

Saliva is a lubricant that helps in chewing, swallowing, and speaking; hence the glass of water often provided for a public speaker whose mouth may become dry from lack of saliva as a result of nervousness. Saliva also helps to cool food when it is eaten too hot, and to dilute irritating substances. Each day about two pints are produced; the flow depends upon the salivary glands, the usual stimulus to secretion being the sight, smell, or thought of food. The glands lie just in front of the ear (the parotid glands, which are swollen in mumps) and under the lower jaw (submaxillary and submandibular glands).

A dry mouth is a natural effect of nervousness. Dryness of the mouth also happens during a fever, from lack of water, and in certain diseases such as diabetes. Some drugs taken for stomach complaints (antispasmodics), for raised blood pressure (hypotensives), and for treating depression may also make the mouth feel dry.

An increased flow of saliva may be caused by irritation from inflamed gums or new dentures. It is sometimes noticed during pregnancy or in a person with a nervous upset. Occasionally the mouth suddenly and unexpectedly fills with clear tasteless salivary fluid (waterbrash). This is sometimes associated with indigestion caused by an ulcer.

WHEN BAD BREATH IS A PROBLEM

Bad breath (halitosis) may be due to septic teeth, food debris between the teeth, inflammation of the sinuses, or disease of the lungs. The cause then is obvious; the teeth are seen to be decayed or unpleasant phlegm (sputum) is coughed up. Usually an unpleasant odor has nothing to do with this type of trouble. Certain products given off during digestion of food pass through the liver to the lungs and are then breathed out; the smell does not signify disease. One example is the breath after eating onions, for the smell of onions comes from the bloodstream through the lungs and continues long after the onions have been digested and absorbed. Garlic rubbed into the soles of the feet can later be detected in the breath!

Bad breath is a nuisance, though seldom a sign of disease. Often only others notice it. If the cause is not obvious, removal of teeth or tonsils in the hope of curing it should be avoided. Those who complain of bad breath but find it difficult to convince others of it are usually suffering from a neurosis. Worry about the imaginary smell can even become an obsession. Even when unpleasant, the breath is unlikely to disturb others except in close contact. Cigarette smoke on the breath can be particularly offensive to a nonsmoker. Often bad breath is just temporary and disappears. Tablets containing chlorophyll are sometimes used, for this is thought to absorb the odor, but there is no scientific evidence for this. Otherwise aromatic substances like peppermint can be sucked to disguise it.

ODD TASTES

The taste of food is appreciated more by the sense of smell in the nose than by the taste organs on the tongue. This is why appreciation of tastes often disappears when one has a cold. Many patients complain of unusual tastes, and no explanation—foul teeth or obvious disease in throat or nose—is found. These tastes, especially when described as metallic or constantly bitter, are usually due to neurosis and other nervous symptoms may be present.

THE TONGUE: AN UNNECESSARY CAUSE OF WORRY

Some people look into their mouths when they feel unwell, searching for signs of disease. For example, they study their tongues in the mirror each morning—like looking at a barometer—and become concerned about coating and other minor changes. This causes more worry than it is worth.

Coating or furring of the tongue, once regarded as a sign of ill health, is common in healthy people and is merely due to thickening of the skin covering it. Coating occurs when mainly soft food is eaten, as on a milk diet, for normal chewing breaks off the old surface cells. Smokers and those who breathe through their mouths at night frequently have coated tongues, but this is nothing to worry about in itself.

Taste buds are prominent at the back of the tongue, and clefts, called fissures, may cross its surface. Some people who get anxious when they notice these, not understanding that the things are normal, may have to be reassured by their doctors. The back of the tongue may occasionally look brown or black. This is partly because taste buds become long and darkened; it is harmless and usually causes no symptoms. The term "geographical tongue" is used when the surface looks like a map where areas of the superficial skin break off and leave islands with irregular borders. This comes and goes for no apparent reason and is often unnoticed, but if it causes discomfort soothing lozenges can be sucked before eating. A more important sign is when the entire surface looks smooth and glazed from loss of taste buds (glossitis), for this may indicate anemia or vitamin deficiency. Little ulcers that come and go are just a harmless nuisance.

TROUBLE WITH GUMS

Inflamed gums (gingivitis) are caused by irregular and crowded teeth, neglect of the toothbrush, tartar on the teeth, and badly fitting dentures.

In pyorrhea the gums are inflamed and bleed easily when touched; sometimes yellow pus can be squeezed out and later teeth become loose. This may, when advanced, cause an unpleasant taste or bad breath. Dental treatment is necessary.

ULCERS IN THE MOUTH

An ulcer on the gums may be due to badly-fitting dentures; these heal quickly when the cause is removed. If a single ulcer or lump persists for longer than three weeks, medical advice should be sought. Occasionally, this may be an early cancer which can easily be cured if treated early.

Recurrent little ulcers are a common nuisance in the healthy and are harmless. People of any age, and especially middle-aged women, may get them. They begin as minute blisters and are painful, particularly when eating or drinking. Crops may come and go for no apparent reason, though some may follow worry. No cause has been found, so no cure is available. Victims of these ulcers may need to be reassured. Soothing anesthetic lozenges (from the pharmacist) can be sucked before meals. Special cortisone tablets sometimes hasten healing and are prescribed by a doctor.

Inflammation of the mouth (stomatitis) can result from irritants like highly spiced foods, too much alcohol or tobacco, and poisons. Antibiotic tablets, especially when sucked, may cause a sore mouth and tongue.

THE GULLET

The gullet (esophagus) is a hollow muscular tube about 9½ inches long, leading from the throat (pharynx) to the stomach. The lump of chewed-up food (bolus) is propelled downwards by a pumping action called peristalsis which operates throughout the digestive tract: a ring of muscular contraction passes downwards and pushes the bolus before it. Peristalsis enables a person, if he so wishes, to eat or drink while standing on his head, a feat that would be impossible if food dropped into the stomach by gravity alone.

The lining of the gullet, in contrast to that of the stomach, has no protection against acid, so gastric juice damages it. Reflux of acid from the stomach into the gullet is prevented by a special valve. If this were not so the life of a trapeze artist, for example, would be impossible as her mouth would fill with stomach contents whenever she hung upside down. The valve works because the gullet enters the stomach at a special oblique angle. When pressure in the stomach rises, as after a big meal or a pint of beer, the end of the gullet is compressed sideways and thus closed. This is also the way the salivary ducts enter the mouth; were it not so, a trumpet player would inflate his own salivary glands every time he played a tune.

DIFFICULTY IN SWALLOWING

Difficulty in swallowing is a feeling of food or drink sticking in the gullet. This may be due to spasm or narrowing of the inflamed gullet, as happens in hiatus hernia because of acid reflux. There is a condition called cardiospasm in which the lower end of the gullet fails to relax and to let food enter the stomach. This is treated by dilatation or operation. Occasionally, in older people, difficulty in swallowing is the first sign of a growth, so the symptom should be reported to the doctor immediately.

The feeling of a lump in the throat is different, for it often occurs in high-strung people, especially in people with worries. Other nervous symptoms like choking feelings, fatigue, and headaches may be felt. This is called *globus hystericus.*

Sometimes it is difficult for the doctor to tell the difference between true difficulty in swallowing and this nervous lump in the throat. For example, one middle-aged woman complained to her doctor that she could not swallow properly. He said to her, "Madam, it is the change" (meaning the menopause). Investigations showed that he was wrong, though in another sense correct. She had swallowed some coins—change given to her when shopping—and these had blocked the gullet. She had done this deliberately and was suffering from mental instability.

DIGESTION

The stomach is a reservoir which, like an elastic bag, adapts itself to different-sized meals and amounts of liquid. Solid particles of food are dissolved by the enzymes and hydrochloric acid of gastric juice, which is about as acid as vinegar, and the early stages of digestion start. Small amounts of liquefied food are pumped at regular intervals from the stomach into the outlet pipe (duodenum). There the acid is neutralized by squirts of alkaline juice from the pancreas. Bile from the liver also mixes with it. Then, in the small intestine, carbohydrates, fats, and proteins are broken down into simple substances which are absorbed, dissolved in the blood, and circulated to the body for growth, energy, and warmth.

INDIGESTION

Indigestion (dyspepsia) usually denotes discomfort, pain, "wind," or a feeling of fullness in the abdomen associated with eating or drinking. Patients often use the wind to cover a multitude of symptoms including heartburn, waterbrash (a tasteless or sour fluid in the mouth), or difficulty in swallowing.

Some common causes of indigestion are stress and emotional upsets (nervous indigestion), ulcers, hiatus hernia, some medicines, and gallstones. Unusual causes are cancer of the stomach, Crohn's disease, and pancreatitis (inflammation of the pancreas).

Investigating the Cause of Indigestion

Indigestion in some patients can easily be diagnosed from their symptoms. Others may need to have a barium meal x-ray. The patient will have fasted overnight, then drinks a glass of barium solution. The room is darkened so that the outline of the stomach can be seen on the x-ray screen. The patient has to be tilted slightly, head down, to permit study of the upper stomach, especially when hiatus hernia is suspected.

Another method is by fiber-optic tubes which are swallowed, allowing the gullet, stomach and duodenum to be seen clearly, photographs to be taken, and biopsies (painless) taken so that small fragments of tissue can be examined under the microscope. The examination is usually performed in an outpatient department; the patient's mouth and throat are made numb and usually an injection is given so that there is little awareness of the examination.

Occasionally the gallbladder may have to be x-rayed. This again causes little discomfort. A special powder, swallowed in a capsule, concentrates in the gallbladder so that it can be seen by x-ray. Some type of fat is given after about half an hour to make the gallbladder contract and to see whether stones are present or not.

Food and Digestion

Many sufferers from stomach trouble have wrong ideas about the digestion of food. These notions may be encouraged by advertisements for patent medicines. For example, patients with indigestion complain of what they call "acidity." But nearly everyone produces acid, which is needed to digest food, and even if there is more acid than usual there are no symptoms. Nor, indeed, are there symptoms with lack of acid. Estimation of the amount of acid in the stomach in someone who considers himself a martyr to acidity may show no acid at all! Nor is discomfort after "acid" food or drink due to acidity, for substances like orange juice are less acid than gastric juice itself.

111

Some foods are traditionally accused of being "indigestible." That there is no truth in this can be proved by taking from the stomach samples of a meal while it is being digested. Indigestion has nothing to do with faulty digestion of food: all foods are digested the same way, and the digestive juices do not discriminate between tough steak and lightly boiled egg.

The point of giving a "light diet"—as during a fever—is to tempt the patient to eat. So many foods are regarded as indigestible—according to folklore rather than fact—that one of these can be eaten almost every day, and it may then be unfairly blamed for discomfort.

Some patients with ulcer or gallstones notice discomfort or pain after certain foods—usually those containing fat. This does no harm, but as it is unpleasant such foods should be avoided. When someone finds that many different foods "upset the stomach," he or she is more likely to be suffering from nervous indigestion than any disease of the stomach itself.

A Touch of Wind

Wind or flatulence is often considered by patients to be a sign of indigestion. Some even believe that the wind which they bring up by burping is due to fermentation in the stomach— a sort of marsh gas generated because what they eat is not being digested properly. However, food cannot normally ferment in the stomach because the acid gastric juice prevents it; the wind that is brought up is nearly all air.

What happens to cause someone to suffer from wind is:

1. The person makes his or her own diagnosis that sensations such as fullness or discomfort are due to wind.
2. He or she tries to bring up and get rid of this "wind"— usually imaginary—by belching.
3. As nearly everyone swallows before a belch, a mouthful of air is swallowed because the mouth is empty.
4. Air therefore gets down. Much is held in the gullet and brought back with a loud report, but some may enter the stomach.

5. Air in the stomach may distend it and temporarily relieve any spasm causing pain.
6. A habit of swallowing air and belching develops and may itself cause more trouble than the original discomfort.

Wind which people belch up is odorless except when mixed with the aroma of recent food. This flavored belch may then mistakenly be regarded as another sign of indigestion. Generally, the feeling of being filled with gas is imaginary, and this can be shown by an x-ray. Sometimes air passes through the intestines and causes rumbling and gurgling (borborygmi) on its way before being discharged from the rectum as wind.

Burping, though many devotees consider it one of the most satisfying of human experiences, should be stopped. It may just be a nervous habit. Sometimes excess saliva in the mouth due to irritation from ill-fitting dentures has to be swallowed, and air goes down as well. Or discomfort (perhaps from inflammation in the gullet or from an ulcer) may be misdiagnosed by the patient as due to wind. He may then start trying to bring up the so-called wind, which will only make it worse.

Most people are cured by an explanation of what happens. If it is a habit, a cork or empty pipe placed between the teeth will help, for swallowing is impossible with the mouth slightly open, though any air comes up naturally. This should be done after meals, when air swallowing is more likely. Peppermint water or an alkali indigestion tablet can be taken instead of belching to relieve discomfort.

HIATUS HERNIA

This causes indigestion because the one-way valve between the gullet and the stomach fails to work owing to a weakness of the hole (hiatus) through the diaphragm, which allows a small bit of the stomach to slide upwards into the chest (a hernia); the oblique angle which helps to form the valve is then lost.

Gastric juice can then flow into the gullet and inflame it, causing heartburn. This is most likely to happen when bending, as in housework or gardening, when in bed, and during sexual intercourse. Sometimes food comes into the mouth as well. Heartburn consists of a hot burning feeling behind the breast bone (sternum). It is different from the warm feeling that occurs when drinking hot liquids, as it usually lasts for a few minutes and is relieved by an alkali such as bicarbonate of soda, which neutralizes the acid. Sometimes hiatus hernia starts at birth, but usually symptoms appear in middle age. Hiatus hernia is quite common in otherwise healthy people and may never cause trouble.

The symptoms may disappear if the patient sleeps with raised pillows or raises the head of the bed to prevent acid entering the gullet during the night. Obesity and tight garments around the waist must be avoided as these increase abdominal pressure, but dieting is unnecessary unless weight reduction is indicated; food should always be chewed thoroughly. Operation is seldom needed.

PEPTIC ULCER

The term peptic ulcer includes an ulcer whether it is in the stomach (gastric ulcer) or duodenum (duodenal ulcer). Both cause indigestion. Duodenal ulcer is more common than gastric ulcer, and is especially frequent in young and middle-aged men. It varies in size from a pinhead to a fingernail, and it is surprising that anything so small can cause so much pain. Pain is felt in the upper abdomen, usually after meals. Sometimes hunger pain occurs and this is relieved by food. The patient is sometimes awakened at about two a.m. by pain, and will drink warm milk to relieve it. The pain is caused by acid irritating the ulcer, so anything that neutralizes acid, whether food, milk, or alkali (tablets or powder), relieves it. The same applies to vomiting, as this gets rid of the acid. Occasionally, the ulcer gets bigger and deeper and complications (perforation or hemorrhage) may follow, though fortunately these are unusual.

Cause of Ulcers

The cause of peptic ulcer remains a mystery in spite of much research. Worry is often blamed and some think that duodenal ulcer is the penalty of stress and even the sign of a successful businessperson. Duodenal ulcer has indeed become common in this century, and it is flattering to think of our society being under greater strain than others during the world's history. Different types of stress have different effects on the body, and the perpetual frustration of everyday life may be more significant than single calamities such as famine or plague.

However, although worry can upset the stomach, little evidence supports the idea that a duodenal ulcer is caused by the strain of certain styles of modern living, for it occurs in anyone from business executive to farm laborer. A slight increase is found in those in responsible positions, such as businesspeople and doctors, but these groups are also more likely to have an x-ray so it is more likely to be diagnosed. Nor does the "ulcer personality"—someone with drive and ambition—always typify an ulcer patient. So worry and stress and strain are unlikely to cause an ulcer, but may make an ulcer worse once it has developed.

Men are more likely than women to get ulcers, though after the menopause the risk is equal. Occasionally ulcers run in families. An ulcer is not caused by any particular food, irregular meals, poor teeth, or alcohol.

Treatment of Ulcers

The aim of treatment, until research reveals the cause and opens the door to cure, is to relieve pain and let a normal life be enjoyed. This is usually possible, and an operation is only required in about ten percent of all patients. Attacks of indigestion (dyspepsia) from an ulcer come and go for no apparent reason, and ulcers tend to heal whatever is done, provided they have not been present for too long. This makes it difficult to assess a new treatment, as anything taken when the ulcer is starting to heal is likely to get the credit for the improvement.

Food helps to neutralize acid and so to relieve pain. Pain can be relieved by altering eating habits, in particular by small meals taken frequently. Ordinary food should be eaten but if any food does cause pain, it should be avoided. No food or drink can actually harm an ulcer, even though it causes pain. In acute attacks, some people are helped by drinking milk about every two hours.

Ulcer patients must eat properly, especially those with a gastric ulcer, as poor nutrition may be a contributing cause. A mid-morning and mid-afternoon snack, and something last thing at night, are advisable. Obesity is a hazard of this way of life, so alkali tablets or powder (available from pharmacists) between meals may be preferable to snacks.

Alkalis are chemicals, in either tablet or powder form, which neutralize acid; they relieve pain by temporarily reducing acid. Alkalis are prescribed to take between meals and when pain occurs, but there is no point in continuing them when the indigestion has disappeared. A vast number of remedies are advertised with a claim that they "cure" indigestion. The essential ingredient of most of them is one or other form of alkali, and as none has been proved to be better than another, there is no need for the sufferer to rush after every new "cure." It is better to find a suitable one and keep to it. A new group of drugs has recently been developed called the H_2 receptor antagonists. Instead of attempting to neutralize acid, these block its production and should help in treating patients with duodenal ulcer.

Trials have shown that gastric ulcer heals sooner in those people who reduce or stop smoking cigarettes, and the same probably applies to duodenal ulcer. No one has conducted a trial concerning alcohol, but as this stimulates the production of acid, it should be avoided while the ulcer is causing trouble, or be taken only after eating.

NERVOUS INDIGESTION

Indigestion (dyspepsia) is often caused by worry. We have learned that emotion can upset the stomach. A sudden shock may make someone "sick with fright" or cause a feeling that the "stomach turned over." Patients with nervous indigestion may have anxieties—a woman worried about her forthcoming marriage or about her work—but often no obvious worry is found. Symptoms sometimes come on after stress and may resemble an ulcer, yet x-rays show nothing abnormal.

Typical complaints are wind, discomfort, foods "lying on the stomach," burning sensations, sick feelings (nausea), "butterflies in the stomach," dislike of wearing clothes touching the skin, and even vomiting. Although the appetite may be all right, feelings of fullness start after a few mouthfuls and the meal has to be stopped. "Sensitivity" to food develops and victims become introspective about eating, thinking that various and occasionally every type of food and drink upsets them— believing that they have a "delicate stomach." Actually, the thought that certain foods cannot be digested is wrong: digestion could be proved to be quite normal by taking samples during digestion through a stomach tube.

Other nervous symptoms may be present: fatigue, irritability, headaches, and sleeplessness. Occasionally indigestion is the bodily manifestation of an anxiety or depressive state which may need the help of a psychiatrist: everything becomes an effort, mountains are made out of molehills, exhaustion prevents even simple activities, and the zest goes out of living. Some patients do not realize how common nervous illness is and how incapacitating it can be; nor that the greater the number of symptoms and the more continuous the trouble, the more likely the diagnosis is to be a nervous condition, and not organic disease.

The cause for the discomfort or pain is usually a tightening or spasm of the muscle of the stomach—similar to what others experience from their colon, called colon spasm. The stomach and bowels normally contract to pump the food along the alimentary tract. This movement (peristalsis) can, if more marked than usual, cause pain and rumblings. Also, if someone is high-strung and anxious the gut may become more sensitive to stimuli that make it contract. A tranquilizer or drug to relax the spasm may be necessary.

The person is cured if a cause for worry can be found and removed, but often the reason may lie hidden in the unconscious mind. A thorough examination and x-rays may reassure sufficiently to cure. A normal diet should be taken, otherwise food fads develop and multiply, and some people may even become dietary invalids. Alleged allergy or sensitivity to certain foods usually lies in the mind and not in the stomach. "Eat what the hell you like" was the advice given by one distraught general practitioner (a man of charm and equanimity, who otherwise never used violent language) to a woman who was obsessed with what she ate. This wise counsel could be proffered more often.

STOMACH UPSETS

The term is used to cover various symptoms: nausea, vomiting, discomfort, diarrhea, and so on. Occasionally they are due to food poisoning or to a virus; medicines are common offenders. Migraine causes vomiting, but there is headache as well.

Food itself, except for gross overeating, seldom causes any upset. Indeed, the capacity of the stomach to digest so many curious foods and to tolerate such insults as alcohol is remarkable. The lining (mucosa) of the stomach produces a special mucus as a protection. Gastritis is sometimes used to explain indigestion which is not serious and for which no other cause is found. This is nothing to worry about, and the diagnosis is sometimes given to those who are really suffering from nervous indigestion. In older people, a large meal may have to be avoided late at night as it can cause hearburn during the night.

The liver is often blamed unfairly, because liver disease seldom causes stomach upsets. "Liverishness" is a vague term for feeling unwell and has nothing to do with the liver.

Hangover

A hangover after a night's heavy drinking is essentially a chemical inflammation of the gullet and stomach. It causes nausea, vomiting, loss of appetite, headache, abdominal discomfort, depression, and sometimes remorse. These symptoms are due to acute alcohol poisoning and whether the cause is gin, beer, or wine makes no difference. The acute inflammation of the upper gut fortunately subsides without permanent damage, in contrast to chronic alcohol poisoning which causes liver damage (cirrhosis) that is often fatal.

Hangover is a self-limiting disorder seldom requiring more than a period of abstinence from alcohol. Some believe in strong coffee; but others find that drinking a pint of hot water in which a teaspoonful of bicarbonate of soda is dissolved helps them to feel better.

LIVER, GALLBLADDER, AND PANCREAS

The liver is a complex factory which plays a vital part in the running (metabolism) of the body. It handles essential ingredients reaching it from the gut after the digestion of food, and prepares them for storage or release into the bloodstream. It detoxifies drugs and poisons. Bile is secreted continuously by the liver but is stored in the gallbladder to be injected into the duodenum during a meal. It is essential for digestion and acts on fats like a detergent.

A block in the system of tubes (bile ducts) conveying bile from the liver to the gut causes jaundice. The skin becomes yellow and the urine goes dark because of increased bile being excreted through the kidneys, but the bowel movements go pale because the bile, which makes them dark, cannot reach the gut. Prolonged jaundice may produce itching (pruritus) and depression. Jaundice can be caused by gallstones (obstructive jaundice), inflammation of the liver (hepatitis), some drugs (especially tranquilizers), hardening of the liver (cirrhosis), destruction of red blood cells (hemolytic jaundice), and growths.

Gallstones

Gallstones may cause pain or discomfort after eating. They sometimes leave the gallbladder and block the narrow bile ducts leading to the duodenum, the patient then suffering from severe pain and developing jaundice. The gallbladder, especially when it contains stones, may become inflamed (cholecystitis) and give rise to pain and fever but often no jaundice.

Why gallstones form is not clearly known. Bile is a concentrated solution of many salts, including cholesterol, so crystals may form and develop into a stone, especially if there is infection of the gallbladder. Gallstones are more common in women, especially those who have borne several children. They increase in frequency with age and are thought to be more common in the overweight and in sedentary workers.

Gallstones occur in about twenty-five percent of those over forty and frequently cause no symptoms. Therefore gallstones, especially if discovered incidentally, may just be left as they are. Sometimes an operation to remove the gallbladder and stones is necessary; this leaves the person fit and able to eat anything. Gallstones cannot yet be got rid of except by operation, though they sometimes pass through the bile duct into the gut and then out of the body. It is possible to dissolve certain gallstones by bile salts, but this is not yet of practical benefit to the patient as treatment has to be lifelong and is not always successful. Claims to remove them by large doses of olive oil and other remedies are false; a lump like a gallstone may appear in the feces, but the gallstones stay in the gallbladder.

THE LARGE INTESTINE

The large bowel (colon) is a reservoir for retaining waste so that this can be discharged at times convenient to its owner rather than at random. Food residues reach the colon about four hours after a meal and can be stored for twenty-four hours or longer. During that time they are dehydrated and changed into a semisolid mass (feces) which is formed into the usual shape by contractions of the colon. The rectum is usually empty, and the reflex which causes the bowels to be opened (defecation) is started off by body wastes entering it; this gives the warning to visit the lavatory. Protection against soiling clothes is provided by the valve at the outlet, aptly described as the "sentinel of social security."

Gas is formed in the large bowel by bacteria which normally inhabit it and feed on insoluble food residues such as cellulose. Everyone expels this wind from the rectum—up to 500 ml in twenty-four hours. Alteration in the odor or volume of the gas does not mean that there is anything wrong with the bowel but is sometimes related to the type of food eaten.

Constipation

Most people indulge in a certain amount of self-medication; the list is headed by medicines taken for moving the bowels. These are called purgatives, laxatives, or aperients, and when more drastic, cathartics. People take them because they are constipated, because they think they are constipated, or because they want to prevent themselves from being constipated. A belief in the purifying properties of a purge has existed since ancient times. It is nonsense, but many people still harbor this idea when they take a laxative or give one to their children.

Constipation means a delay in passing feces which may be harder than usual. It does not cause ill health, just unpleasantness in moving the bowels and perhaps a sense of fullness in the rectum. It is quite wrong to think that constipation means not having a bowel movement every day. Some people do have a bowel movement every day, some twice a day, but other healthy people just move their bowels three times weekly or even less. Claims are made for periods up to eighty days and longer without moving the bowels, the holder of such a record remaining fit with a good appetite and plenty of energy. In the past people believed that poisons of some sort were absorbed into the bloodstream if the bowels were not moved daily, and that these caused bad breath or headaches. However, no toxins or poisons from the movements are absorbed or cause any of these symptoms. If anyone does get a headache with constipation, it is due to the rectum being distended, and not to poisoning.

Astronauts move their bowels only twice weekly because space food contains no residue. It is also natural for the bowels not to be moved when a person stops eating, such as during a fever or after an operation, when days may pass without the desire to move the bowels. The only precaution is that the elderly and debilitated have to be watched to make sure that feces do not accumulate in the rectum. Temporary constipation may be caused by an emotional upset or by a change of routine when traveling. Then a single dose of a mild laxative may be worthwhile, just to start the normal reflex going again. If constipation arises unexpectedly in older people, a doctor should be consulted as it may be the first sign of obstruction due to inflammation or a growth.

The most common form of constipation is partly due to the rush of modern life: the call to go to the lavatory is ignored so that a bus or train may be caught. The rectum then fills with body wastes and the signal for the reflex that controls emptying no longer works. Other reasons for neglecting the urge to go to the toilet are laziness, a cold or dirty lavatory, false modesty, or painful piles. Vacations make people forget because they have other interests or because there is a line for the john, and it is this and not a change of water that causes constipation!

The reason that some people become addicts to laxatives is because they start with the idea that a daily bowel movement is essential for keeping fit. This wrong idea has been encouraged by advertisements designed to sell laxatives. The reader is made to think not only that a missing bowel action is serious, but also that symptoms of being "run down" are due to this. The lay-person easily accepts this, for purgatives have been regarded as a cure for many illnesses from early times.

Diarrhea

Diarrhea means that movements are loose and visits to the toilet more frequent. There are many different causes: infection, nervous tension, drugs, or growths. If diarrhea does not subside within a week or two, it should be reported to the doctor.

A sudden attack of diarrhea and vomiting may be due to food poisoning, especially when several people are affected at the same time. It starts within twenty-four hours of eating contaminated food and disappears after a few hours or days. All that is usually necessary is rest and plenty of fluids (soft drinks, weak tea or coffee, and so on). Antibiotics seldom help. Many foods convey germs, but most suspect are those foods which lie around after being handled, as germs multiply inside them, particularly in hot weather. Prepared meat dishes, pastes, meat pies, artificial cream, trifles, salads, and unwashed fruit are particularly suspect. Germs often reach food from the feces of the person handling it, so food poisoning would almost be wiped out if everyone washed their hands after going to the lavatory. It is thus very unfortunate that washing is still not possible in some public lavatories. Safer foods are those where handling is likely to be minimal or where germs have been destroyed by cooking—tinned foods and freshly cooked fish and meat, for example. If the cleanliness of the water is suspect, bottled drinks can be used or water chlorinated with a tablet obtained from the local druggist. Water from the hot tap is safe, providing that the water has been really hot and so sterilized.

Irritable Colon

Irritable colon (colon spasm or colon neurosis) is a common complaint causing diarrhea and discomfort in the lower abdomen, especially on the left side. The large bowel no longer stores and dehydrates movements properly because it is sensitive and easily goes into spasm due to stimuli that do not affect a normal bowel. Sometimes this spasm causes griping pains and constipation instead of diarrhea as it holds up passage of body wastes. Occasionally severe pain is felt in the rectum.

Irritable colon is a nuisance, though never serious. Often it is partly nervous, like migraine. The bowel acts like a mirror in reflecting the worries and stresses going on in the mind—a fact sometimes noticed by the victim. Anxiety or fear may prolong symptoms. It is frequent in intelligent and conscientious people who are otherwise healthy and not particularly high-strung. Some become too conscious of their bowels and how often they are moved, and they complain of constipation, meaning that it is necessary to take a laxative or enema in order to obtain a bowel movement that satisfies them. If asked how long they go without a bowel action, a typical reply is "I never let my bowels go more than a day without a movement." Such an individual may be dissatisfied with the amount and appearance of the movements—which may resemble those of rabbits—lamenting that his bowels do not move enough. Occasionally, his whole life becomes centered round the bowels, and it is difficult to cure this obsession.

Diarrhea usually occurs only in the morning and does not wake the patient at night. Patients are sometimes told that they have inflammation of the colon (colitis). This is misleading, for the colon is not inflamed and it is nothing to do with conditions like ulcerative colitis. Most sufferers respond to reassurance, especially after investigations have excluded serious disease, and doctors may also prescribe antispasmodic tablets. Bowel action in the healthy varies between three times daily and three times weekly, and it is not necessary to move the bowels each day. Sufferers should be reassured that the size and shape of their stools depend upon the amount of water mixed with them and in any case do not matter. Most people live a normal life in spite of their sensitive bowel, and many are cured by a diet high in fiber.

The Problem of Piles

The Chinese proverb that nine out of ten men have piles is an exaggeration, but piles (hemorrhoids) are a common and harmless condition. They are dilated normal blood vessels at the anus. Like varicose veins, which they resemble, they sometimes run in families.

Piles either cause no trouble or occasionally hurt or bleed, especially when torn by the hard stools of constipation. Other conditions, such as growths, occasionally start with bleeding so the doctor should be consulted. Pain from piles only occurs when a complication such as prolapse or clotting (thrombosis) arises; pain occurring when moving the bowel may be due to a split, called a fissure, in the skin next to a pile. Itching (pruritus) may be due to piles but is more often caused by some other harmless disorder. Piles seldom need treatment, though constipation should be avoided by the adoption of a high-fiber diet. Only occasionally do they have to be dealt with by injection or operation.

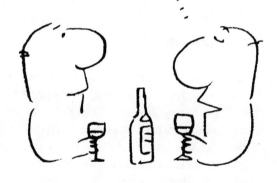

Here's to the fight against addiction!

chapter 7

DON'T GET ADDICTED

Any weekday afternoon a fat, wheezing man may be seen walking down the steps from one of a hundred restaurants. His eyes bulge, his face is purple, and the whiff of alcohol on his breath is mingled with smoke from a large, half-smoked cigar in his right hand. In no sense would he consider himself ill. He might admit he was a little too fat, but he likes his food; he might say that it would be sensible for him to smoke less; he might agree that, like other people, he occasionally drinks too much, but he would not see himself as an alcoholic nor does he believe he is likely to become one. If someone were to say to him: "If you did not eat, smoke, and drink so much you would live longer," he would reply: "The future you advise for me sounds so awful it would certainly *seem* longer." This capacity for self-deception lies at the heart of the problem of addiction to tobacco, alcohol, or drugs.[1]

ADDICTION TO ALCOHOL

There are, of course, problems in defining illness and unhealthy behavior, partly because there is so much individual variability in the response of the body to long-continued use of a drug. We would describe anyone who drinks two bottles of whiskey a day as ill, saying he was an alcoholic: he is dependent on alcohol and his illness is alcoholism. If we were rabid teetotalers we might say that someone who drank one glass of sherry a day should not do so, but we would not define him as ill, nor would we say that this was likely to lead to ill health in the foreseeable future. So what should be said about the millions of people whose consumption of alcohol lies between these extremes?

A useful definition of alcoholism is that it is "the intermittent or continual ingestion of alcohol leading to dependence or harm." This definition cuts out drunkenness, which is acute

[1] See *How Much is Too Much?* Stanton Peele, © 1980 Prentice-Hall, Inc.

intoxication. It comprehends *urge* (compulsion, craving), actual *withdrawal symptoms* (such as tremor), and *harm,* whether to the individual or to others. The aim of this definition is to state the least that all sufferers from alcoholism have in common. Any one of the three features described (two of dependence and one of harm) is enough, if it is a consequence of regular drinking. It is also useful to think of an *alcohol-dependence syndrome* (with dependence or addiction) as well as of disabilities, which can be either related to or coexisting with the syndrome. The essential elements of the alcohol-dependence syndrome include a narrowing in the variety and type of drinking behavior; increase of drink-seeking behavior; increased tolerance to alcohol; repeated withdrawal symptoms; repeated relief or avoidance of withdrawal symptoms by further drinking; subjective awareness of a compulsion to drink; reinstatement of the syndrome after abstinence.

Incidence of Alcoholism

There has been a steady increase in the amount of alcohol consumed in the past thirty years, so it is likely there will be continuing increases in rates of alcoholism. Consumer expenditure on alcohol has risen over the past ten years; for example, in England over five times as much money was spent on beer in 1975 as in 1960.

Spending varies within different income brackets: the greater the household income, the more money is spent on alcohol, despite the fact that manual workers spend proportionally more of their income than do people in other occupations. Between 1965 and 1975, the U.S.A. consumption of alcohol nearly doubled. In that period admissions to hospital for alcoholism, drunkenness convictions, and convictions for drinking and driving rose dramatically. Similar increases in deaths from cirrhosis of the liver and alcoholism have occurred, and among executives the death rate from cirrhosis is 22 percent higher than the average for the population—perhaps a reflection on the wider availability of alcohol consumed during business lunches, sales conferences, and so on. All these figures continue to show a steady increase. In recent years there have been increases in the number of women alcoholics, but the ratio of men to women is still of the order of four to one.

Effects of Alcohol

The effect of alcohol on the central nervous system is, of course, the primary reason for its widespread consumption. The central nervous system is more markedly affected by alcohol than any other system in the body but, contrary to the layperson's view, alcohol is a primary and continuous depressant of the nervous system. Stimulant properties have been attributed to it because those under its influence often become talkative, aggressive, and overactive. Apparent stimulation arises from the unrestrained activity of parts of the brain freed from inhibition as a result of depression of the inhibitory control mechanisms.

While the exact pharmacological mechanisms of the action of alcohol remain controversial, we do know that its behavioral and depressant effects are dependent on the amount taken. The first consistent changes in mood and behavior appear at blood levels of about 50 mgm (milligrams) percent. The majority of individuals feel carefree and released from many of their ordinary anxieties and inhibitions. As the blood alcohol rises, more functions of the brain are affected. Clumsiness and emotional changes follow from a level of 100 mgm percent, and at levels of 200 mgm percent those parts of the brain which control movement and emotional behavior are measurably impaired. At a concentration of 300 mgm percent, the great majority of individuals are quite obviously severely intoxicated. Thereafter more primitive areas of the brain are increasingly depressed. Confusion and then progressive stupor and anesthesia follow, and a killing concentration lies betwen 500 mgm percent and 800 mgm percent.

The behavioral effects are more marked when the blood

alcohol is rising. Blood alcohol levels are affected in various ways. For example, if alcohol is greatly diluted with water, absorption is delayed, and when alcohol is taken after food lower blood alcohol curve peaks are found. The rate of disappearance of alcohol from the body varies slightly between people and even in the same individual from day to day or from hour to hour. A very large person taking the same amount of alcohol as a small person would have a slightly more rapid fall in body alcohol. An average individual (154 pounds) disposes of alcohol at a rate of about two-thirds of an ounce (9 ml) an hour. Heavy drinkers may have a greater degree of tolerance to the effects of alcohol.

Interaction with Other Drugs

Alcohol is a powerful pharmacological agent with widespread effects, and may interact with other drugs. Such interactions are moşt likely to occur following continuous heavy drinking, but even moderate drinking may constitute a risk with some medicine. Some commonly seen drug-alcohol interactions can be predicted on the basis of the known pharmacological properties of alcohol. For example, as alcohol is a central nervous system depressant it may potentiate the effects of sedatives, including the barbiturates and benzodiazepines (Librium, Valium, or Mogadon). When an overdose of barbiturates is taken in conjunction with alcohol the resulting coma may be deeper and more dangerous.

Alcohol and Mood

Alcohol removes unpleasant mental feelings, which is one reason why people drink. The easy availability of a tension-relieving drug makes it unrealistic to expect people not to use it to relieve tension. Much unrealistic health education has been directed at telling people not to use alcohol for this purpose; there is no evidence that drinking a couple of glasses of sherry at the end of the day in order to unwind is likely to lead to any harm. Many people without serious problems in life adjustment use alcohol occasionally or regularly simply for pleasure or as a minor tranquilizer. Some people with larger or more constant trouble with their feelings use alcohol for apparently similar reasons, and it is they who are at risk. Some of them may at first drink regularly because of social pressures, but will later continue to use alcohol for its mood-changing effects.

Alcohol is not a good drug for dealing with unpleasant or uncomfortable feelings of any serious proportion. Because alcohol is a drug to which tolerance develops, the likelihood is that alcohol will gradually be needed in larger and larger quantities. Not only does drinking then begin to fail in its original purpose of relieving psychological distress, but it actually begins to make matters worse. Heavy drinking itself produces symptoms, and the person concerned may misinterpret these as evidence of a condition which requires further drink to put it right.

Alcohol in large and continued quantities produces a very depressing effect on mood, and the person becomes prey to all sorts of doubts, miseries, suspicions, and general gloom. An acute fear of particular situations may develop. Heavy drinking leads very easily to a state of mental distress which not only the subject himself is likely to misinterpret but which a doctor can misdiagnose as "depression" or "anxiety" if the drinking story is withheld. Treatment with antidepressants or tranquilizers will be ineffective, and may well worsen the situation. Anyone who drinks because of "nerves" should ask whether these "nerves" are due to drinking.

Personality and Alcoholism

Two personalities have been singled out as prone to excessive drinking. One lacks self-confidence, has little self-esteem, and may even at times be disgusted with himself. Such a person may have been deprived of affection in childhood, or been frankly neglected or mistreated. Self-punitiveness is a characteristic of such drinkers, apparently long pre-dating the onset of addiction. Alcohol may give respite from mental self-flagellation as well as from a pervading sense of insufficiency and inferiority.

The second, very different, type of person is free of self-loathing and is not troubled in personal relations but is the self-indulgent individual who may have been pampered in childhood. Such a person can find difficulties in the realities of work. Personal relations and marriage may add up to a bleak list of obligations and responsibilities. These may be met more or less effectively, but this person may also discover that drinking can confer an episodic mental vacation. When under the influence of alcohol happy, perhaps exciting, daydreams can be summoned to transform mundane existence.

Prolonged continuous drinking also exerts effects on personality. An alcoholic may be a hostile person whether it is apparent or not. Aggressive emotions, like dependent needs, may become expressed with drinking. Some people who are normally gentle become enraged when drunk. Some alcoholics resort to physical violence or they may turn their anger against themselves when they become depressed.

An alcoholic may loathe himself and describe himself with utmost contempt as rubbish. Each day is full of defeats. It may be that he drinks and impairs his ability at times when demands are placed on him, with the result that he does not meet expectations. The shame and disappointment of behavior in performance can then be reduced by more drink, the only drawback being that performance is further impaired.

Society and Alcoholism

Society now recognizes alcoholism as a major social and health problem, and alcohol appears recently to have replaced drug addiction as the focus of public concern. However, it is doubtful whether alcohol is seen as a drug in the same way that heroin, for example, is regarded as a dependence-producing substance. Society still remains somewhat ambivalent about alcohol—which is both a recreational beverage and a dependence-producing drug. Nevertheless there are certain aspects, such as the effect drinking has on driving and on certain families, which have stimulated the increased attention now being paid to alcohol.

In 1974 one in three drivers killed in road accidents had blood alcohol levels above the statutory level. Between 10 p.m. and 4 a.m. on weekdays the proportion of driver fatalities with blood alcohol concentration over the legal limit rises to 51 percent, and on Saturday nights to 71 percent. In a survey of 2,000 road accidents a drinking driver was involved in 25 percent, and his or her alcohol consumption was deemed to be a major factor in 9 percent.

The adverse effects of drinking on the family are obvious when matters have reached extremes. A survey of Alcoholics Anonymous members showed that 35 percent of men and 28 percent of women who went to AA believed that drinking had broken up their marriages. Excessive drinking may contribute to violence in marriage, and in a study of a hundred battered wives fifty-two of the victims reported that their partners engaged in frequent heavy drinking.

The minor manifestations, however, require a more sensitive eye for their detection. The man or woman who is drinking heavily is likely to be perceived by the family as someone who has failed as a breadwinner, and this may produce a permanent or intermittent sense of strain and deprivation. They may also be seen, in many ways, as failing to fulfill ordinary family obligations.

Treatment for Alcoholism

Reviews of the literature and treatment of alcohol dependence show that claims for the efficacy of specific treatment and treatment regimes have outrun the evidence. The value of any of the wide range of specific treatment methods still has to be incontrovertibly demonstrated—what was effective might well be the rather nonspecific influences of support, under-standing, exhortation, and education. Alcohol dependence should be viewed as a chronic relapsing illness.

Hospital care may be necessary when alcohol is with-drawn, as there may be withdrawal symptoms which require specialized medical treatment. Disulfiram (Antabuse) has been used for over thirty years, and patients who continue to take it have a better prognosis than those who stop the drug. Citrated calcium carbumide (Abstem) is another drug which can be used to help some patients who wish to remain abstinent, but have difficulty in doing so. Both drugs have no effect when taken by themselves but when taken with alcohol produce an unpleasant reaction. For this reason they can be helpful to someone who wants to abstain from drinking completely (because of alcohol-ism) but finds this difficult because of social obligations or craving. Aversion treatment has also been used but there is still uncertainty as to whether conditioning has much to offer. Group therapy for alcoholism has been widely used and Alco-holics Anonymous is a valuable supportive organization, although only a minority of people who are encouraged to join AA in fact do so.

Recently attempts have been made to train some patients to return to limited drinking rather than to aim at total absti-nence. It has been known for many years that it was possible for a small number of alcoholics to return to controlled normal drinking, but many workers in the field found this difficult to accept. For the majority of alcoholics total abstinence remains the best goal for treatment.

How Much is Too Much?

Treatment of alcoholism is at present of limited value, and attempts at prevention must therefore be taken seriously. One of the factors in the development of dependence of any type is availability, so consideration should be given on how to control this. There is no consistent relationship between reported consumption of alcohol and the appearance of "problems" until people admit to having drunk more than an approximate average *daily* consumption of just over eight single whiskeys or two quarts of beer. Above this point there is a marked acceleration in the reporting of problems resulting from drinking. The total alcohol consumption in a population has a direct bearing on the number of people with alcoholism, to the number of deaths and illnesses associated with alcoholism, and to alcohol-related problems. This favors the view that alcohol-related problems increase as a result of liberalizing alcohol control measures. Taxation policies have been shown in many countries to affect total consumption and also the incidence of *delirium tremens* and chronic alcoholism.

In Denmark, for example, relatively higher taxes on distilled spirits and lower on beer led to a temporary change in drinking habits with a decrease in the occurrence of the physical illnesses of chronic alcoholism. In Finland, where the number of sources for the purchase of alcohol has recently been increased, *per capita* rates of alcohol consumption have similarly increased.

In England the Erroll Commission, which studied the alcohol licensing laws, considered alterations which would permit longer hours for the sale of alcohol. While this might benefit the tourist industry, the possible social implications of such a change have recently been under scrutiny. If increasing the opportunities for the sale of alcohol means increased consumption, then any such changes should be looked at not only from an economic standpoint but also from that of their possible effect on health in the community.

Health authorities are not usually in a position to advocate the use of revenue controls as a public health measure, while those responsible for taxation do not usually consider the prevention of illness to be one of their functions. Nevertheless, more consideration might be given to the public health consequences of such methods of indirect control, including, for example, additional taxes on alcohol, changes in the times during which alcohol may be consumed, changes in the number of facilities for its sale, and controls on sales to minors.

GUIDE TO ALCOHOL CONSUMPTION

Alcohol is a weakly addictive drug and has to be taken regularly over a long period of time for harm to develop. As a rough guide the following table may be helpful.

Average Daily Consumption

Milliliters of Absolute Alcohol	Single Whiskeys		Light Wine (Bottle)	Pints of Beer		Result
0	0		0	0		Teetotaler
30	2			1		No harm
60	4	or	½	2	or	No harm
90	6			3		No harm
120	8	or	1	4	or	Some harm
150+	10+			5+		Alcoholism

Rough Equivalents

1 shot (single) whiskey	45% alcohol content
1 sherry glass sherry	20% alcohol content
1 wineglass light table wine	10% alcohol content
½ pint average beer	5% alcohol content

(All these contain 15 milliliters absolute alcohol)

ADDICTION TO TOBACCO

When are tobacco smokers ill? In the United States millions of people smoke, and we can hardly say that they are all ill. Many of them are addicted to the nicotine in tobacco, but addiction by itself does not constitute illness or the majority of the population would at some stage find themselves declared ill. There is, however, plenty of evidence to show that smokers are more likely to develop numerous diseases later in life.

Dependence on alcohol, tobacco, and other drugs can cause severe health problems, and so can overeating. Because of the very widespread use of tobacco and alcohol the amount of ill health caused by these socially acceptable drugs still greatly exceeds that caused by misuse of other dependence-producing substances. Treatment of dependence is of limited effectiveness and seldom adequately evaluated. Prevention is desirable, though difficult to accomplish. Because of their wide-spread use, the socially acceptable drugs (tobacco and alcohol) lead to the greatest number of casualties in terms of both dependence and harm.

During the past twenty-five years many studies have clearly shown that cigarette smoking is a major cause of diseases and premature death. It has been estimated that in the United States any adolescent who smokes two cigarettes will have a 70 percent chance of being a regular smoker for the next forty years. Sir George Godber put forth again in 1978 the statement he made when he was Chief Medical Officer of the British Department of Health and Society Security. He said:

> In previous reports a very conservative figure of deaths associated with cigarette smoking has been used, but this year [1972] an attempt has been made to calculate more closely the total mortality related to cigarette smoking, of which little more than a third is due to lung cancer. On reasonable assumptions about the main groups of such deaths from lung cancer, chronic bronchitis, and

ischaemic heart disease, some 80,000 premature deaths probably occur in England and Wales each year and for the whole of the United Kingdom the number must approach 100,000. Of course a high proportion of these deaths occur in older people, but there are enough in the working age groups up to sixty-five to mean that the premature deaths before that age cause each year the loss of 190,000 man years of working life. We cannot estimate the amount of working time lost from illness due to cigarette smoking but it must be responsible at least for the greater part of the 38.6 million days of sickness absence certified as due to bronchitis in 1969. . . . The benefit to health of abolition of cigarette smoking would be enormous, and economic advantage from the prevention of lost working time and the reduction of the cost of the health care required to relieve the ravages of the habit would certainly add up to many hundreds of millions of pounds each year. This is no harmless indulgence but the biggest single avoidable menace to health in contemporary life in Britain causing, all told, perhaps ten times as many deaths as do road accidents and nearly as many deaths as all the cancers unrelated to smoking put together.

Smoking and Health

The diseases associated with smoking include coronary heart disease, lung cancer, chronic bronchitis, and emphysema. More than half the adult population smokes, but the present trends do indicate a reduction in the number of men smokers in higher social classes. Those who do smoke are smoking more, and the number of women smokers is increasing. The reports by the Physician General on smoking and the hazards to health, along with government tax increases, have all contributed to some reduction in cigarette smoking.

In the United States several pounds of tobacco is smoked per adult per year. This includes all types of tobacco, in cigarettes, pipes, and cigars. Over 90 percent of all tobacco smoked is in cigarettes, about 5 percent is pipe tobacco, and 3 percent cigars and cigarillos. The last has almost doubled over the last few years. A large proportion of smokers smoke filter-tip ciga-

rettes. The male adult smoker smokes on average twenty cigarettes a day and the female fifteen cigarettes a day, with
both men and women between the ages of thirty-five and
fifty being the heaviest smokers. Restrictions on advertising
and the government warning on cigarette packages would appear to have had little or no effect on cigarette consumption.
The publication of the tar and nicotine content of cigarettes has
enabled the smoker to identify the content in different brands
of cigarettes, and to switch to a low tar brand.

There has been wide publicity on the dangers and health
consequences of smoking following many official U.S.A. reports
and the large prospective study of doctors by Sir Richard
Doll and his colleagues, which convincingly showed that smoking is associated with a number of serious and preventable
diseases. These reports convinced the majority of doctors to
stop smoking, and others have also stopped. Smoking withdrawal clinics may have helped some, but there is little knowledge of why some people are more successful in giving up
smoking than others. The number of cigarettes smoked, the
inhaling of smoke, and the age at which smoking is started are
important contributions to mortality. In a study of British
doctors twice as many smokers as nonsmokers were found to
have died before reaching the age of sixty-five. An association
was clearly shown between cigarette smoking and lung cancer;
when doctors reduced their cigarette smoking by half, their
death rates from cancer of the lung were reduced by one-third,
while in other men in the population aged thirty-five to sixty-
four years who continued to smoke the death rates from lung
cancer increased by a quarter.

Tar (a carcinogen) is the distillate from cigarettes; when a
cigarette is smoked it acts as an irritant and can produce
malignant changes in the respiratory systems of animals. Many
heavy smokers have microscopic changes in the bronchi which
are caused by an irritant or irritants, and these are believed to
be precursors of malignant changes. It has been estimated that
90 percent of all cancers of the lung are caused by smoking.

Deaths from chronic bronchitis are two-and-a-half times more common in heavy smokers, and it is estimated that in half the deaths from bronchitis smoking was a major cause. Many deaths from pneumonia and heart disease are associated with chronic bronchitis or emphysema in men between forty and fifty years of age. Smoking causes coughing, breathlessness, and increased production of phlegm. In young adults these effects disappear when smoking is stopped, probably as a result of lung elasticity, but continued smoking plus smoke inhalation may lead to permanent lung damage and finally to chronic bronchitis and emphysema.

Death rates from coronary heart disease are about 50 percent higher in smokers than nonsmokers. Deaths from coronary heart disease in middle-aged men who are heavy cigarette smokers are four times higher than among nonsmokers of the same age. Cigarette smoking is a risk factor, and is independent of other factors such as high blood pressure and raised cholesterol in the blood. Both disability and sick leave from work are higher in smokers than nonsmokers. It is estimated that 38 million working days are lost yearly due to bronchitis, and of these 28 million are the result of smoking. Other effects of cigarette smoking include delay in healing (for example, in cases of peptic ulcer), decay of gums, and dental loss. Women who smoke during pregnancy have babies who weigh less than those of nonsmokers and they miscarry more frequently.

In summary, cigarette smoking frequently causes death at an earlier age and is also responsible for a very large amount of disability in men and women. This is a loss not only to the smokers themselves but also to their families and to society, and makes considerable demands on expensive medical care.

Smoking as an Addiction

Nicotine can, like alcohol and other drugs, cause dependence: there is a pharmacological effect which strengthens the tendency to use cigarettes. There are more similarities between drug dependence and alcoholism than there are differences.

First there is the matter of dependence. The smoker, like the future alcoholic or opiate addict, begins to use cigarettes confident that he or she will not become addicted. People begin to smoke largely to satisfy curiosity, to conform to the expectations of friends or associates, to achieve a certain status among these peer groups, or to express disregard for the social norms of society. Particularly among young people there is a strikingly high correlation between the reasons for taking up smoking and the reasons for taking up other forms of drugs.

With tobacco smoking, the initial motives of curiosity, conforming to the behavior of family and friends, or rebellion against authority are soon reinforced by the effects of the drug nicotine. With each cigarette the pharmacological effect strengthens the tendency to continue its use. Each repetition of the behavior weakens the likelihood that motives for nonuse can modify the developing pattern of drug use. Many investigators now believe that with tobacco (nicotine), as with other drugs, there eventually comes a time for many users when the abrupt cessation of use causes a distinct and characteristic pattern of behavior that is specifically and immediately alleviated by using nicotine.

Once this state develops, relief from abstinence becomes a new source of reinforcement for the drug-using behavior. The tobacco withdrawal syndrome is shorter and less distressing than opiate or alcohol-barbiturate withdrawal syndromes; however, the effect of nicotine in inhaled cigarette smoke wears off so rapidly that the user must replenish the body's supply several times an hour. Tobacco smoking shares with other forms of drug use the likelihood that both drug and withdrawal effects can be conditioned to certain cues. Long after a smoker or alcoholic has been abstinent, common stimuli may elicit a craving, very much like that which was once produced by acute withdrawal of the drug. For example, a person who has stopped smoking may think of the pleasures of a cigarette when he or she has a cup of coffee, and may find it particularly difficult to resist a cigarette proffered at a party.

Social Acceptability

A second factor in the pattern of nicotine use is social acceptability. In some respects tobacco use is unlike all other forms of compulsive drug use. Smoking is still so socially acceptable that the concept of nicotine addiction or compulsive tobacco use is only just beginning to emerge. With alcohol there is a distinction between those who use the drug occasionally, in socially appropriate situations, and those whose use of alcohol is inappropriate, injurious, or excessive: alcohol use is socially acceptable but problem drinking or alcoholism is not.

In contrast, people who smoke cigarettes are not generally expected to apologize or to try to curb the habit, except in public places such as train compartments for nonsmokers, or the homes of nonsmokers. The general public hardly recognizes the idea of tobacco abuse, and does not yet have a concept of nicotine addiction. Most people feel no sense of shock or dismay when public figures, elected leaders, actors, or sports heroes smoke in public. The motivating force of a society that has a definition of how much is too much tobacco has not yet come into being. Those who would give up smoking do so mainly out of concern for their own health and well-being. In the U.S.A., with the growth of the nonsmokers' rights movement and the climate of people's rights in general, many people are considering more carefully where they smoke, but public opinion has not yet reached the point where people will feel motivated to give up the habit solely because it is socially unacceptable.

Is Nicotine so Important?

There are many people for whom the unique relaxing, yet also alerting and irritability suppressing, effects of nicotine may be extremely useful in helping them cope with the frustrations of a complex society. Despite this view of the usefulness of nicotine some people are concerned about placing too much emphasis on a safer cigarette. It may be true that the effects of nicotine have made tobacco universally used and some may find these effects more pleasing or more necessary than other people. Yet at the same time one cannot help but be impressed with the fact that a few years ago about 66 percent of doctors in England and the U.S.A. were cigarette smokers and that now only 25 percent are still smoking. Since no one believes that the practice of medicine has become less frustrating or less stressful over the last decade, one can only conclude that at least half of the physicians who once seemed to need nicotine now function without it.

Does Treatment Help?

Some 18 percent of smokers become ex-smokers. This so-called natural discontinuance tends to occur after thirty and increases with age, especially after sixty, and the majority of this group who give up smoking do not find it difficult. On the other hand, among those who continue to smoke nearly half would like to stop but are unable to do so. Health, expense, and social pressure are the most important reasons for wishing to stop. There is no evidence that any drug or psychological treatment exists which has any advantage over simple, supportive counseling to guide a smoker through withdrawal from tobacco and in relearning to function efficiently and contentedly without smoking. There is essentially no specific treatment for those who wish to abandon tobacco.

The medical profession provides a good example of the possibilities and limitations of health education. Doctors who, it must be assumed, know more of the hazards and dangers of opiates than comparable non-medical professional groups, nevertheless have much higher rates of opiate dependence than comparable groups in the general population. This example illustrates that availability appears to be a more powerful factor than knowledge. On the other hand, smoking habits of doctors have changed markedly, and in some countries the number who are cigarette smokers has been halved, apparently as a result of their professional knowledge of the risks to health. It is said that the most effective health education message was one that was run a few years ago with the message: "200,000 doctors have stopped smoking. Do they know something that you don't?"

Anti-smoking campaigns directed specifically at young people have been carried out using radio, movies, and television; suggesting that smokers are sexually unattractive was thought to be one promising approach. However, long-term evaluation studies of anti-smoking propaganda to schoolchildren suggest that it has not been very successful, and when followed up there appeared to have been little or no long-term change in smoking.

Compulsory abstinence enforced by government is not likely to work, but there are various other actions which might bring about some changes in the future. Health education, anti-smoking advertisements, films, posters, and leaflets are already part of an effort to dissuade people from smoking; alternative methods also need to be explored and monitored. Marked increased taxation on tobacco is unlikely to result in a sudden dramatic change in consumption rates, but might have long-term effects on premature mortality and disease. Cigarette advertising controls could be more stringent; less attractive packaging and the abolition of coupons might also help. Tobacco sales, particularly to children under sixteen years old, could be curbed. Removal of licenses following the proved sale of tobacco to children might act as a deterrent to store owners, provided that this was enforced. Changes in the amounts of tar and nicotine in cigarettes might all gradually lead to less (and less harmful) smoking.

A safer cigarette is needed. A totally safe cigarette would be one which would provide the same death rates and illnesses for people who smoked as for those who had never smoked. A "safe" cigarette might be a "safer" cigarette if the death rates were lowered, even if they were not as low as among non-smokers. Many smokers who cannot give up smoking would like to switch to a safer cigarette, if it produced the same effects as their usual brands without the serious health consequences.

ADDICTION TO OTHER DRUGS

Sedatives, hypnotics, tranquilizers, stimulants, anti-depressants, and analgesics are capable of producing a state of dependence in people who take them repeatedly in sufficient dosage. The use of drugs to produce sedation, oblivion, elation, or euphoria is endemic in most parts of the world. These forms are often long-established by custom and tradition. They are regulated and stabilized. Their dependence production is low and often they are preparations with minimum risk.

Epidemic outbreaks have to be distinguished by such factors as rapid spread, lack of previous social experience, and explosive outburst—the introduction of gin in the seventeenth century, the use of amphetamines in Japan, or marijuana smoking by young people in the last decade would be examples. With improved communications and increased travel there have been recent examples of the spread of the use of drugs previously confined to certain areas, for example, alcohol from the West to the East and marijuana from the East to the West.

The patterns of misuse of drugs have been changing rapidly, and a recent report pointed out that in all countries there has been an upsurge in the number of people dependent on drugs that has attained the dimensions of an epidemic. Most of the drugs concerned are hypnotics or tranquilizers, but the list includes antipyretic analgesics, central stimulants, and marijuana (dependence on opiates seems relatively low). In general, six trends are discernible in drug dependence: a growing incidence in young people; new patterns in drug dependence (for example brain stimulants, administered intravenously); a rapid increase of the abuse of well-known drugs in other age groups (sleeping drugs, antipyretic analgesics, and central stimulants); a rising frequency of multiple dependence; an increasing number of women dependents; and a rapidly increasing problem of alcoholism.

Causes of Addiction

There are many possible causes leading people to become dependent on drugs. This may be a manifestation of an underlying character disorder in which immediate gratification is sought in spite of the possibility of long-term adverse consequences and at the price of immediate surrender of adult responsibilities. It may also be a manifestation of delinquent-deviant behavior in which there is pursuit of personal pleasure in disregard of social convention (so that to some this is primarily a moral problem). Drug dependence may also arise from an attempt at self-treatment by persons suffering from psychic distress as a reaction to social or economic stress, frustration, or blocked opportunity; or the more persistent problem of depressive illness, chronic anxiety, or other psychiatric disorders; or physical illness or a belief that a drug has special powers to prevent disease or to increase sexual capacity.

There have been changes in the use and misuse of drugs in this country in the last ten years. The most noticeable change is a lessening of morbid interest in the phenomenon. Although the number of people trying illegal drugs has increased, the concern about drug dependence as a problem has decreased, and concern about alcoholism as a problem has become much more noticeable. The current pattern of drug dependence appears to be that there is a small increase which is spread over the country as a whole so that some areas which have previously had no drug misusers now have a few.

Barbiturates and Other Sedatives

Another recent change has been an increasing concern with the question of whether barbiturates are useful drugs or not; a consensus appears to be forming that there are other drugs which can be used in their place in the treatment of mild anxiety and insomnia. Although the danger of drinking combined with the taking of "sleeping pills" is well-known, and the dangers of addiction are known to doctors, barbiturates are still very widely available. Most of the concern about barbiturates is not because of physical dependence on them but because a large number of people take overdoses of barbiturates when subjected to stress or unhappiness. In some areas 10 percent of all admissions to general hospitals are of patients who have taken such overdoses.

Studies on the functioning of the nervous system suggest that all these drugs act in a similar manner to alcohol. It is not generally recognized that the sedatives can produce almost exactly the same sequence of behavioral dangers as alcohol, because they are normally used under different circumstances. They are most commonly taken at bedtime, under conditions where a minimum of stimulation from the environment normally occurs, and as a result the depression of the arousal system by the action of the drugs leads rapidly to the onset of drowsiness and sleep.

If these drugs were taken in a similar social setting to that in which alcohol is normally used, they would produce the same sequence of changes seen with alcohol. There would be a gradual reduction in the degree of environmental control over behavior and an increasing freedom of expression. This type of effect is fairly common among people who use barbiturates and other sedatives regularly during the day.

One important difference among barbiturates and other sedative drugs relates to the rapidity, intensity, and duration of the effect of the dose given. Phenobarbital has a slow onset of action and acts for a long time, which makes it very suitable for prolonged, even sedation or for the control of epilepsy. At the other end of the spectrum are drugs such as pentothal, which has an extremely rapid onset of action, intense effect, and very short duration, and because of this is given almost exclusively for anesthesia.

Between these two extremes are drugs such as pentobarbital (Nembutal) and amylobarbital (Amytal, Tuinal) which have a fairly rapid onset, intermediate duration, and a less intense effect; they can be used for modifying the mood, and the dosage given does not necessarily put the person to sleep if there is no desire to sleep. These differences are very important, as they determine which barbiturates and sedatives are likely to be used for both medical and non-medical purposes.

Worry about Sleep

People worry about insomnia and many people report that they sleep badly. It is not uncommon for people in these circumstances to take drugs in an attempt to sleep better. In general the drug treatment of insomnia is fairly useless. The reason for this is that when people take sedatives over a period of time tolerance develops. In other words they have to take more of the same drug to obtain the same effect. At the same time that tolerance develops they develop slight dependence on the drug so that when they stop taking the drug symptoms appear. When a sedative is given for a short time it makes a person drowsy; if it is given for a longer period it has little effect, but when it is stopped he is more than usually alert and restless. If a person regularly takes a sedative for a month, withdrawal symptoms can be shown when the sedative is no longer taken, by means of electroencephalographic studies during sleep. If someone is sleeping badly and is regularly taking drugs the best thing to do is to reduce gradually and then stop all the drugs. This will make sleep worse temporarily, but eventually the normal pattern of sleep will be regained and sleep will be better.

Everyone sleeps less as they get older, and the majority of people wake in the morning feeling tired, seedy, and without energy. It is probably better to call this middle age and learn to live with it than to seek a magic tranquilizer to remedy it. A glass of warm milk is probably the best night sedative.

Tranquilizers

The term *tranquilizer* applies to a wide variety of different chemical structures. These have different primary effects but have in common one important property: a relatively much greater suppressing effect on emotional reactions to stimuli than on the general level of alertness. This makes them differ from the alcohols, barbiturates, and other sedatives. The selective effect upon emotional reactions is probably produced in an area of the brain known as the limbic system.

The "major tranquilizers" which are used in the treatment of severe mental illness include chlorpromazine (Largactil) and other similar drugs. These appear to have little or no direct inhibitory effect upon the arousal system, and some may even stimulate it slightly. In theory a drug which has no effect on the state of alertness but markedly relieves emotional tension or distress should be a ready candidate for widespread non-medical use. However, most of these drugs are slow in onset or have rather unpleasant side effects on blood pressure and motor coordination if given in large doses to relieve tension. Because of this the major tranquilizers have had little or no appeal for non-medical users seeking an immediate short-lived change in mood.

The "minor tranquilizers" such as meprobamate (Equanil), chlordiazepoxide (Librium) and diazepam (Valium) are closer in action to barbiturate and alcohol. As might be expected, they are often used in a very similar manner. They are among the most widely prescribed drugs in all of medicine. Some people use them for short-term effects in exactly the same way as they would use a few alcoholic drinks, and the problems of dependence upon the minor tranquilizers have become well recognized in the last few years. Complications associated with their long-term use are similar to those associated with long-term use of barbiturates or alcohol.

Amphetamines

Amphetamines are central nervous system stimulants. Their effects include wakefulness, a sense of well-being, lessening of fatigue, and a feeling of increased energy and self-confidence. They also reduce appetite, and for this reason they were used in the past for treatment of obesity. In excessive doses there may be restlessness, rapid speech, inability to sleep, euphoria (an exaggerated sense of well-being), irritability, tension and anxiety, aggression, slurred speech, staggering gait, rapid and irregular heartbeats, dry mouth, and tremors of limbs. The development of abnormal thinking and delusions and hallucinations of a persecutory kind may also occur. There are also other effects on the body due to stimulation of the sympathetic nervous system. Blood pressure is raised, and dilation of the pupils, relaxation of the smooth muscle of the gastro-intestinal tract, the urinary bladder, and bronchioles of the lungs occur with the secretion of thick saliva.

The danger of misuse of amphetamines was not fully understood until some twenty years or so after their introduction into medical practice. The social consequences of amphetamine dependence include illegal acts to obtain the drug, deteriorating work record, disruption of family life, amphetamine psychosis, and a tendency to aggressive behavior. Originally those abusing amphetamines were often middle-aged, overweight persons with depression, or those who had ready access to drugs (doctors, nurses, pharmacists), and at one time they were widely misused by young people. However, the overall amount misused has probably decreased in the past few years.

Cannabis, Marijuana, "Grass," or "Pot"

Cannabis is a mixture of substances. Of the scores of chemical compounds that the resin contains, the most important are the oily cannabanoids including tetrahydrocanabinal (THC), which are the chief cause of the psychic action. Reactions to the use of cannabis vary and are influenced by the behavior of the group using it. Sensations can become more vivid, especially visual ones, and contrast and intensity of color can increase although there is no change in acuity. Euphoria occurs, though not invariably, with giggling or laughter that may seem pointless to an observer, and the size of objects and distance may be distorted. Time as experienced may appear longer than clock time—thus a subject asked to say when sixty seconds has elapsed may respond too early, and if asked to say how long some period of time was, overstates it. Sense of time can disappear altogether, sometimes leaving a distressing sense of timelessness. Recent memory and selective attention are often impaired.

Cannabis continues to be used fairly widely by young people (and an increasing number of the middle aged) though many more have experimented with it a few times than use it very regularly. It has ceased to be a source of great concern, and the heated debates of earlier years recommending either increasing efforts to stamp out its use or alternatively decreasing penalties have died down. Few people now believe that it definitely causes cerebral atrophy, but even fewer believe that it is a safe drug. Concern should now be concentrated on the effect of cannabis on such skills as driving, and the fact that until recently there have been no simple and reliable tests to confirm its use.

Hard Drugs

The use of the highly dangerous drugs commonly grouped under this heading, including cocaine, heroin, morphine, LSD, and so on, still remains fairly small in the U.S.A. However, the use of cocaine is growing among some groups of upper-class or upper-income business people. There are special clinics for those who have become addicted, and treatment is available through private and public agencies. It is probably safe to assume that few addicts can be numbered in the executive stream of the population. Unless the addiction was rapidly controlled they would not remain in senior positions for very long. They may encounter the problem in their adolescent children, but that problem falls outside the range of this book.

ADDICTION TO GAMBLING

When people gamble, money is the usual stake, and it is often assumed that the motivation underlying gambling must be related only to this. However, this may be no more than a means to an end. The money may be used to purchase something else, such as excitement, amusement, or comfort. Risk-taking itself can be pleasurable. If the uncertainty continues for a limited time, as is the case in gambling, the feelings of tension that are associated with it may be relieved when the uncertainty is ended. The beneficial effects of this experience were referred to by the ancient Greeks as *catharsis*; in many cases it may be this element that makes gambling so attractive.

Among those who gamble there are some who do so to a greater extent than average, in terms of either the amount of money spent or the time given to the activity. In some of these people, gambling leads to harmful financial, social, and psychological consequences for themselves and their families. In spite of this the gambling continues, and has been referred to as compulsive, pathological, or disordered gambling. These terms are synonymous and tend to be used interchangeably. Although the term pathological originally had a medical connotation it has more recently been used in a broader setting as, for example, in the term "social pathology." It does not necessarily imply that there is an illness underlying the condition.

Pathological Gambling

Pathological gambling can usually be recognized by the presence of one of the following:

1. Concern on the part of the gambler and/or the family about the amount of gambling that is considered to be excessive.
2. An overpowering urge to gamble so that the individual may be intermittently or continuously occupied with thoughts of gambling. This is usually associated with a subjective experience of tension which is found to be relieved only by further gambling.
3. The subjective experience of an inability to control the amount staked once gambling has started, in spite of the realization that damage is resulting from this.

The pattern is similar to those seen in relation to alcohol and drug misuse. In the case of drug misuse every drug produces its own syndrome of dependence. It has been found that the importance of physical factors in drug misuse has in the past been considerably overrated, at the expense of psychological and social factors.

It has been suggested that some types of pathological gambling are due to a state of psychological dependence on the activity of gambling, and that this may be a learned or conditioned response arising out of various personal and social factors. In view of this it is not surprising that the management of pathological gambling can be very difficult.

A pathological gambler is a person who has a high need for risk and who can also be seen as one who spends a large amount of money on the intangible commodity of risk, in a manner similar to that of the collector who purchases expensive items such as antiques. The difference is that an antique is tangible and the collector has something to show for the money spent. The experience of risk in gambling just passes, and there is nothing to show for it afterwards.

Gaming Machines

It is interesting to watch someone using a slot machine, occasionally winning some coins or tokens which become part of the total being staked until all are lost. An apparently fruitless, boring, and pointless exercise, but one now widely practiced.

Slot machines, or one-armed bandits as they are often called, exploit certain simple principles of operant conditioning using a schedule of intermittent reinforcement. Extensive research in both animals and humans has shown that if behavior is rewarded when pursued, a habit is built which must be considered in its own right. If the reward is given intermittently and is unpredictable in its occurrence this process of learning is enhanced as long as the intervals between rewards are not too prolonged. This is even more true if the total rewards over a given period of time remain constant. It has been pointed out that long-term net gain or loss is almost irrelevant in accounting for the effectiveness of this schedule. It is apparent that in slot machine gambling the gambler's responses, which are a product of processes of learning, are predetermined.

When gambling really gets out of control, affecting both work and social life, skilled help is needed, both for the addict and for his or her family (see list of addresses starting on page 211).

ADDICTION TO FOOD

Gluttony is one of the seven deadly sins; obesity is an illness. Illness is hard to define except as an absence of health, but obesity can be found in the Standard International Classification of Disease and it is reasonable to classify it this way because death is one form of absence of health. Overeating may, for some people, become as much an "addiction" as the other things we have discussed.

The risks of being too fat in adult life have been well documented. Overall the mortality of men who are 10 percent or more overweight is one-fifth higher than average. The corresponding increases for people 20 percent and 30 percent overweight are about one-third and two-fifths. In women the risks are slightly less. These increased risks are associated particularly with deaths from diabetes and from vascular disease and coronary heart disease. Being too fat is also linked with increased incidence of other illnesses which do not necessarily shorten life. These include those associated with the mechanical problems of excess weight, including osteoarthritis (damage to joints particularly affecting the weight-bearing joints in the legs, hips, and knees), varicose veins in the legs, and hernias.

Obesity is also linked with raised levels of cholesterol and other fatty substances in the bloodstream. They may account for the increase in gallstones in fat people, and also the link with atherosclerotic disease which affects the blood vessels. This tendency, together with the fact that it is also related to raised blood pressure, could be expected to increase the risk of disease of the coronary arteries. Being too fat throws an extra strain on the heart. It is not simply a question of permanently carrying around the equivalent of an unnecessary suitcase—the heart itself may be too fat and flabby.

Eating is pleasant. Cooking is one of the very few arts that can be practiced daily for a lifetime. Food can be indulged in at will. It is not grossly expensive and one's own overeating does not affect other people (except indirectly if an overweight breadwinner drops prematurely dead). Even small variations from an ideal diet can have striking effects if they are maintained for years. There is no truth in the belief that fat people often eat less than average. It is certainly true that *everyone* can lose weight if they eat less. Obesity is directly linked with the amount of food eaten and its type: fat, starch, and sugar are especially likely to lead to gains in weight. Very large quantities of fat may cause nausea, and its intake is therefore often self-limiting; protein needs more energy to metabolize it, which is why it forms the basis of many slimming diets.

Most people can lose weight for a few weeks, but less than 25 percent can reverse a habitual pattern of overeating and stay slim. The underlying cause of fatness is simple: at some time the body has taken in more calories than it could use, and they were stored. An intake of 100 calories above requirements every day (two slices of bread, a medium-sized boiled potato) may result in a weight gain of 10 pounds a year.

There is one simple, safe way to reduce weight—change the diet. The only reliable way to do this is by changing eating habits in such a way that a new pattern of eating is permanently established. In theory it is simple to lose weight just by eating less, but in practice this can be difficult. Many people have found that joining an organization such as Weight Watchers gives them the extra support which enables them to lose weight successfully.

CONCLUSIONS

Many of the major illnesses that occur before old age are preventable or could be much reduced in incidence by changes in the pattern of our daily lives. Treatment of many of these conditions is dismally ineffective, and prevention is always better than cure or attempted cure. Regular use of many substances can lead to addiction, and while small degrees of dependence may not be very harmful some types of addiction are more harmful than others. Moderation in all things should be the watchword. In an affluent society it is very easy to cause damage by dependence or addiction, when a new and harmful need is created through the excess use of a substance that was originally taken merely for pleasure.

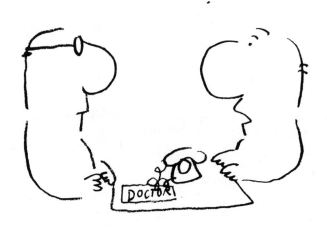

chapter 8
CANCER:
NOT ALL BAD NEWS

There is probably no type of illness that causes more worry than cancer. Even a fear that symptoms might be due to the disease may cause endless anxiety and misery.

WHAT CANCER IS

What is cancer? It is in fact a whole group of diseases, with some features in common—though the differences between them make any single "breakthrough" from research or treatment most unlikely. What all cancers have in common is that they represent a distortion of the normal growth and functioning of one of the cell types somewhere in the body. The abnormal growth may be due to disordered function of the cells themselves or to malfunction of the controlling mechanisms of the body. In its early stages a cancer is commonly no more than a simple growth or swelling—and at that stage removal of the growth by surgery or by treatment with radiotherapy may give a complete, lasting cure. But the unique feature of cancers is their ability to spread, when advanced, to other parts of the body to the point where the vital organs are affected and their functions destroyed.

FEARS ABOUT CANCER

In addition to its medically unique features there is something special about cancer in the effect it has on people's minds—filling them with fear, as if the diagnosis of cancer amounted to a death sentence, preceded by a frightful mutilating operation. Above all, perhaps, cancer—and especially advanced cancer—promotes fear because of the mistaken belief that it is always attended by agonies of pain. These beliefs are found in highly educated and intelligent people; they are emotional in origin and in most instances they are wholly mistaken.

These exaggerations may have been fed by the tradition

of doom written into so many medical textbooks a couple of generations ago when nearly all the cancers *were* incurable; when "heroic" surgeons *did* perform appallingly mutilating operations in their attempts to eliminate the disease as radically as possible; and when the methods available for controlling pain *were* hopelessly inadequate. Awareness of the spectacular advances that have been made in the past twenty years in the control and cure of cancers has yet to percolate through to the public.

Indeed, pessimism about the possibility of the successful treatment of cancer—with which so many doctors were formerly indoctrinated—was transmitted to nurses and hospital staff and is still to be found throughout the community. To an alarming extent the layman's attitude includes fears which are, for several cancers, quite out of touch with reality. One psychological explanation is that the virtual eradication of tuberculosis—a disease attended by many taboos and strange irrationalities—has contributed to the pathological anxieties people so often have about cancer. Cancer may have inherited the psychological and emotional morbidity that was once attached to TB.

PUTTING CANCER IN PERSPECTIVE

It is in fact quite reasonable that a very serious group of diseases which claims the lives of large numbers of people, including young people, should be viewed with fear. It is obviously quite normal to be frightened about cancer. What is perplexing is that nothing like the same degree of dread exists in relation to diseases of the heart and circulation, which cause at least two-and-a-half times as many deaths and are far less easy to treat effectively than many cancers. Even so, it is not surprising that enormous sums of money are spent on research and on methods for improving treatment when one considers that thousands of people die each year in the United States from one form or other of this group of diseases. What is not sufficiently appreciated is that a substantial proportion of these people are in their seventies or eighties and that a great many of them die of cancer without any of the misery that people imagine to be inevitable. Furthermore, many old people on whose death certificates the word cancer appears have in fact died of sheer old age—and in some cases other conditions have been the immediate cause of death. In an aging population it is easy to be misled by figures which seem to suggest that cancers are seriously on the increase. At least a part of the increase (which adds, of course, to popular fears) is due to improved methods of diagnosis and more efficient methods of registration. Only one form of cancer is increasingly rampantly—cancer of the lung—and that is the cancer that is most easily preventable in our present state of knowledge.

While it plainly remains true to say that the cancers constitute a very serious health problem, it does also need to be said, as forcefully as possible, that it is a health problem which is by no means as grim as the majority of people believe. There are very few cancers which remain as resistant to effective treatment today as they were two or three decades ago. The supreme exception, again, is lung cancer—the form of cancer with the worst outlook of all. Lung cancer in both men and women has now assumed epidemic proportions, yet it is an epidemic almost entirely due to excessive cigarette smoking over a long period.

SEEKING A CURE

Lung cancer (and a very few other tumors) apart, cancer is in many instances now curable. It may come as a surprise to most people to learn that thousands of people are fully cured of their cancers every year in the United States. By "fully cured" is meant that these people recover after treatment to the point where they have exactly the same expectation of life as people of the same age and sex who have never developed cancer. For these it can be said, quite legitimately, that they have had an "attack" of cancer from which they have recovered. What is more, there is little doubt that another several thousand at least could be added to this total if only people could be encouraged through information and education to be more concerned about their health and the way they live; if they could learn to look on cancer more realistically so that they would go to the doctor quickly if they notice a persistent change in their normal pattern of health.

When to Seek Advice

Perhaps one of the most tragic examples of the waste of human life is seen in the middle-aged man or woman—perhaps with a young family—who dies prematurely of a cancer that would have been cured if it had been detected and treated early, or at least kept under control for many years of useful life. There is no doubt (from systematic surveys and other studies) that great numbers of people are filled with mortal dread if they discover a lump in the breast, or some bleeding from the bowel. They feel that it *must* be cancer, and the distorted and sinister thoughts induced overwhelm their common sense.

The American Cancer Society puts out the slogan "Don't frighten yourself to death." Sadly, that is exactly what very many people still do. Instead of seeing a doctor quickly, they just hope a lump or some other symptom will go away; or they say that they will have it looked into when the present rush of work is over; or when they have time during their holidays; or when the children are back at school—and so on. The weeks lost by these delaying tactics (caused by fear) may well spell the difference between life and death. And, of course, these weeks are filled with an agony of anxiety which might so easily have been dispelled entirely by a simple test.

At least three out of five lumps in the breast, for instance, are not due to cancer at all and can be dealt with very simply. Often surgery is not needed, but if it is, all that is required is a very simple, small operation which leaves the breast completely intact. Likewise, bleeding from the bowel is far more likely to be due to piles than to cancer. But if either of these symptoms *does* lead to the discovery of a growth, the sooner it is detected and treated, the better the chances of a cure.

There are no characteristic symptoms of the different forms of cancer (and there are many different forms), but there are certain departures from normal health which need prompt attention because they *could* be due to malignancy. For example, the presence of blood in the urine or stools, or unexpected bleeding in women after menopause; the discovery of a lump; an unexplained persistent cough; changes in bowel habits (for instance, alternating constipation and diarrhea); persistent hoarseness of the voice; unexplained and continued indigestion when the alcohol intake and the eating of rich foods have not been excessive; unaccountable loss of weight; the enlargement of or bleeding from a darkly pigmented mole or wart. But it cannot be emphasized too strongly that all these conditions are frequently caused by disorders which are not cancer at all. They may, however, still be serious or troublesome enough to need active treatment—again, the sooner the better.

The lump in the breast and the bleeding from the bowel were given as examples of conditions that *might* be due to cancer but are much more likely to be due to other simple disorders. In the case of the other examples, it is significant that many of them may be caused by functional irregularities due to stress. For instance, everyone is familiar with the nervous cough, the attacks of diarrhea, the nausea and indigestion, and loss of weight in people who are beset with an emotional crisis. Many people in highly demanding work who tackle their responsibilities with commitment, and who have very heavy workloads, are under stresses which reveal themselves not only in the mind and feelings, but in the workings of their bodies as well. It is imperative, however, that those to whom this applies should not allow themselves to attribute these abnormalities purely to overwork and stress: they must be examined properly and without delay.

CANCER OF THE LUNG

Lung cancer tops the danger list—with a five-year survival rate of only about 5 percent following major surgery—simply because there may often be no warning signs at all. However, it cannot be said too often that there is no longer any doubt about the clear causal relationship between heavy cigarette smoking and lung cancer, the incidence of which, though falling off slightly in men, continues to rise sharply in women. The number of new cases in men is still rising at a formidable rate—it is important to realize that only the *rate* of increase for men compares somewhat favorably to the rate of increase in women.

Lung cancer is preventable. Nicotine and other physical, psychological, and social aspects of smoking all contribute very powerfully to this most dangerous addiction. Until our social habits and patterns change profoundly, it is likely that there will be great numbers of cigarette smokers. But it is, of course, possible to hope for changes in social habits, especially by way of education of young people. Among older people, even ones of high intelligence, it is discouraging to realize the power of addiction. One might imagine that the threat of developing lung cancer (to say nothing of the other crippling diseases associated with tobacco) would be enough of a deterrent. But obviously this is not so, and indeed the reaction of many heavy smokers is to reach for another cigarette to steady their nerves.

Against this, it is very encouraging that nonsmokers are beginning to influence the scene—and that the smokers are beginning to accept the efforts being made by pressure groups which have led to the use of fewer smokers' compartments on public transportation and to the proliferation of nonsmoking areas in movies, theaters and other public places. There are already a good many places of work where smoking is forbidden, and the ban is usually accepted by the work force where it is seen to be necessary as a safety measure. Yet "no smoking" is of course a safety necessity for the individual worker, and perhaps much could be done by banning smoking at work through executive decision.

One of the many arguments used by smokers to justify continuing is that they have been smoking so long already that if their lungs have been damaged, it is too late to do anything about it. This is untrue. The effect of smoking is *not* irreversible—even for the person who has smoked heavily for a long time. A long-term study of a large group of doctors who were very heavy smokers years ago, but who succeeded in giving it up, has shown that they can now enjoy the knowledge that their risk of developing lung cancer is steadily falling, and for some has reached the very low level that applies to nonsmokers.

A switch from cigarettes to cigars or a pipe seems to reduce the harmful effects on the lungs, but there is some doubt about the advantage of this strategy for the inveterate cigarette smoker, who is likely to inhale cigar or pipe smoke in the way cigarette smoke was inhaled. (The person who has always smoked a pipe and perhaps the occasional cigar will usually have developed the habit of puffing rather than inhaling.) Even when this is taken into account, it *is* a good idea for any committed smoker to wean himself from cigarettes to a pipe.

For executives (and for everyone else) the right decision is to stop smoking completely. It might be seen as a responsibility of executives to encourage their colleagues and staff to join the ranks of nonsmokers.

CANCER CHECKS

There are, of course, other forms of cancer that can be prevented. In human and personal terms it is just as important for a woman not to develop cancer of the cervix—although the size of the problem in social terms is far smaller. There is no doubt that with full use of the available facilities for cervical smear tests (Pap smears), the hundreds of deaths a year from this form of cancer could be radically reduced. It is therefore most important for the woman executive—however busy she may be—to find the small amount of time needed to have this test regularly. And she too has the responsibility to encourage her colleagues, including junior ones, to do the same.

A pioneer effort of health care on behalf of employees at every level was undertaken many years ago by the British department store, Marks and Spencer Ltd. There can be no doubt that many lives have been saved. In this company a great deal of personal advice and encouragement is given to employees to pay more attention to their health; health checks, including Pap smears, are made by the highly organized medical services of the firm. In organizations that cannot develop facilities of this order, a great deal can nevertheless be done through the initiative of executives to persuade their women employees to make use of the service which is available in many free or inexpensive clinics throughout the country.

The situation is not so straightforward when it comes to screening for breast disease. Although techniques have been developed in a few clinics to the point where they are safe and valuable for the very early detection of breast cancer, this approach to the earliest possible detection is still limited to those who can afford to have it done privately or who may be within range of one of these specialist clinics. Recently in the United States there have been doubts about the wisdom of x-ray screening (mammography) and the National Institutes of Health have recently recommended that regular screening should not be advised for women aged less than fifty unless they are known to have relatives with breast cancer.

An important opportunity does exist, however, in breast self-examination, and explanatory leaflets can be had from the American and Canadian cancer societies. It is, perhaps, too optimistic to expect that any but the most intelligent and emotionally-balanced women will develop the habit of monthly examination of their own breasts. Many start doing it but after a while they give it up. As with Weight Watchers, there is reason to believe that mutual encouragement within a group can greatly strengthen motivation, and this can apply in the case of breast self-examination—if women can be induced to discuss it among themselves. This kind of approach has been shown to increase the numbers who keep it up.

The same logistic problem applies to the provision of precautionary tests for early cancer of the bowel as a national service. The methods used have been improved to the point where such a test is scarcely even uncomfortable, and it is widely used by people of executive status. Cancer of the bowel is much more common in Western countries, where people tend to eat a lot of over-refined foods—and this may well apply especially to executives who are obliged to do a great deal of entertaining. Here again, however, there is still insufficient evidence of the value of the procedure to justify a national screening program.

THE IMPORTANCE OF DIET

The value to health of eating a diet high in fibrous, unrefined foods, or of taking additional bran, has already been described. There is now growing evidence that this hastens the passage of the contents of the bowel to a remarkable degree, and such a diet protects the bowel lining from exposure to potentially dangerous substances that contribute to the development of bowel cancer.

National variation in nutrition may be significant in other ways in connection with cancer. In Japan, for instance, the low intake of fat in the diet has been suggested as a factor in the relatively low incidence of breast cancer in that country. But the different countries, different cultures, and different environments make generalizations impossible. At the present stage, perhaps all that can be said is that cancer, in common with many other diseases, has to do with the way we live. The way many executives live, with excessive and all but unmanageable workloads, may well make them vulnerable to illness. The important question is always the familiar one of priorities. A sick executive has not been doing a good job if he or she is indifferent to the basic priorities of health. One manager, for instance, was always so busy that he forever postponed his appointment with the dentist to adjust his false teeth. Constant erosion of tissues predisposes to the development of cancer in the mouth, and this was the cause of his death—because he was too busy to see his dentist.

ACCEPTING THE CHALLENGE

We pay too little attention to the simple hazards to health. We are inclined to think of people who do so as hypochondriac neurotics. We worry in case it should cause some kind of public panic to talk openly about cancer and the rational steps that can be taken to control it. In biological terms, fear is a cause of inhibition, negativity, and inaction; so it is in psychological terms. A serious illness can be seen as a mortal threat, or alternatively it can be seen, personally and socially, as a challenge. A challenge produces exactly the opposite reactions. The person (or the community) is stimulated to do something about it.

Both in prevention and in the after-care of people who have had treatment for cancer, it is vital to sustain this attitude of challenge. For those who have had treatment there is good reason to believe that their subsequent lives will depend crucially on the care and support of those around them, to help them to meet the crisis as a challenge and not as a threat. The first can result in almost miraculous degrees of rehabilitation and restoration to a full and active life, notwithstanding the handicaps and disabilities that may have resulted from the illness. The other produces depression and demoralization—an open invitation to the disease process to spread and for the person's health to deteriorate.

The Control of Pain

Many people with cancer that has reached the stage of being difficult or impossible to control have as their greatest fear the terrifying expectation of intolerable pain—a fear even greater than that of death itself. They should be reassured. Great advances have been made, quite recently, in understanding and controlling pain. Formerly, doctors and nurses concentrated mainly on the control of acute pain in those illnesses from which recovery might be expected. In chronic pain, whether from cancer or another type of disease such as arthritis, the pain goes on and on unless its characteristics are understood. Very commonly such pain is intensified by tension and anxiety, and if this can be dealt with—as it can—people previously needing massive doses of powerful drugs to keep the pain at bay can be maintained entirely pain-free with properly timed doses of simple analgesics. Under sensitively controlled conditions there are many people who can work and enjoy life to within three or four weeks, or even less, of their deaths. Where this is possible, the executive may have the privilege of making the decision to find the right kind of job to keep a colleague or employee at work, thereby giving him or her the will to go on living, overcoming the feeling of isolation that comes to ill but sufficiently capable people who may feel that they are not wanted.

Such situations may not occur very often. Perhaps of greater importance is the responsibility of the executive to be on the lookout for the member of staff who comes to work looking strained and worried. Of course, this may be due to one of countless causes, but one very important one is the anxiety brought on by the development of a symptom which the person fears may be due to a developing cancer. Bearing in mind the fact that popular attitudes cannot be changed quickly and that the very word "cancer" provokes, for many, the kind of fear we should be trying to allay, it is usually more helpful to encourage the man or woman to have a *health* check rather than a specific *cancer* check.

Caring Concern

Finally, because we should be trying to replace the fear-ridden superstitions about cancer with rational, common-sense attitudes, there is a great opportunity for people in executive positions to arrange the occasional seminar or lecture to keep the subject of health care at work at the front of people's minds. In the case of cancer it is most important that those who lecture have an up-to-date knowledge of the advances that are being made, in order to help both the patient and the family. Leaflets can be obtained from the main cancer charities and from the U.S. Department of Health.

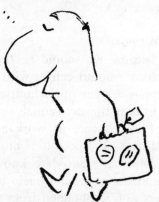

I've got my pills,
my medical insurance,
my thermometer and my
own stethoscope...

chapter 9

THE TRAVELER

When travel by sea to foreign countries took five days to Europe, for example, and as much as six weeks to Australia the stress attached to it was minimal, and the only discomfort might be sea sickness, due to rough weather—and possibly aggravated by too much good living during the many hours that had to pass each day, and the cheap price of drink. Today this sort of travel is impossible for the executive owing to the competitive nature of business and the speed with which management decisions must be made. Executives now travel by air, and this has produced its own new problems. Some are physiological—the much-publicized factor of jet lag; others are organizational—the difficulty of carrying clothes suitable for several climates within a limited luggage weight. The experienced traveler will learn little from this chapter, but others may find something that may help to make their journeys less stressful.

TRAVELING BY AIR

First, what exactly is jet lag? Its cause is the time change inevitable in flights from east to west or west to east. Every country in the world takes noon as the time that the sun is overhead, so local time varies by as much as twelve hours from the time in New York. Each 15° of longitude is equivalent to one hour in time; London to New York represents five hours. The traveler leaving London about midday in a conventional jet, which takes seven hours to reach New York, arrives between 2:00 p.m. and 3:00 p.m. local time—in London the time would be between 7:00 p.m. and 8:00 p.m. If he flies by Concorde he arrives one or two hours earlier than his London departure time. The practical effect is that his day is lengthened by the five hours of the time difference. It is only too easy for him to be entertained by his New York hosts throughout the late afternoon and evening, going to bed at 11:00 p.m. local time, when the time in London is 4:00 in the morning. He will then get into bed and sleep for an hour or two, but his internal clock will wake him at his London time of 7:00 a.m.—only 2:00 a.m. New York time. He will pass a restless night and find he is very tired the following day.

The sensible plan for the transatlantic traveler is that on arrival in New York he should go to his hotel, have a short rest, some fresh air, a light meal and go to bed about 9:00 p.m. (in London 2:00 a.m.), possibly taking a mild sedative. This will give him eight hours good sleep, and though he will still wake rather early he will be refreshed and, which is most important, he will have had sleep when nature intended him to have it.

This example is given at some length to illustrate the time changes that upset circadian rhythms. The body works on a natural twenty-four hour timetable, and many functions—such as the secretion of urine—shut down at night automatically. These rhythms, and the more obvious ones of sleeping and waking, cannot be changed at will, so anyone moving to another time zone finds that his body is still functioning on its usual timetable; if it is 9:00 a.m. in London the body is alert, wanting breakfast, even if it is 4:00 p.m. in India. These rhythms will adapt, of course; it takes about a day to adapt to each change of two to three hours, so after a flight to China or Australia nearly a week will pass before adjustment is complete. None of these changes does any permanent harm; given time, the rhythms automatically adjust themselves. Some of the symptoms that occur may, however, be unpleasant. How can the discomforts be kept to a minimum, with as few problems as possible over sleep, digestion, and mental and physical alertness?

TRAVEL PEACEFULLY

Beginning with the flight, it is wise to remember that airports are tiring, hectic places, and to try to arrive in good time and relaxed. Those who are nervous about flying should consult their doctor, and not be afraid to take a mild sedative for the journey. Long flights are often boring, and because the time passes slowly there is a great tendency to overeat and to drink too much alcohol—especially if it is free. Ideally the traveler should eat light meals at his regular home time if the meal arrangements on the flight make this possible. This is not so important on a seven-hour flight, but someone flying to the Far East, for example, may otherwise find himself eating a three-course meal at four in the morning.

In a modern jet passengers are pressurized to about 5900 feet; smokers should try to reduce consumption as much as possible. Carbon monoxide is absorbed from tobacco smoke, and at this cabin pressure the amount in the blood may be doubled. Some exercise should be taken; experienced air travelers get up and walk the length of the cabin from time to time, to prevent any swelling of the ankles.

Probably the most important thing is the maintenance of fluid balance. Pressurization tends to dry the air, and it is only too easy for passengers to become partially dehydrated. This process does not have to be corrected entirely with whiskey or gin and tonic; plenty of fruit drinks or water should be taken as well, and noncarbonated drinks are preferable to soda water or other carbonated drinks. Drinking more than average quantities of fluid particularly applies when the traveler is flying to a hotter climate.

If these simple measures are followed there is no reason why a flight of seven hours or more should impair physical well-being. The functions which are most likely to be upset are sleep, digestion, and bowel action. Most people still have a somewhat disturbed sleep on the second night, waking rather early, and a night sedative may well be a sensible precaution. The third night will in all probability be quite normal.

Allow for Brain-Drain

The most important effect of changing time zones—which has been proved in several experiments with elaborate psychological tests—is some impairment of the powers of thought and opinion-forming. Mental acumen is considerably (though temporarily) dulled; the jet-lagged traveler behaves as if he had been drinking: he may well be loquacious and quite euphoric. Clearly, then, a businessman should not arrange for a meeting to be held immediately on arrival, especially if he would normally be asleep at this time. Ideally the traveler should arrange to have one day off for a five-hour time change, and two days off for a ten- or twelve-hour time change. It is therefore a considerable advantage to arrive on Saturday, and hold the meeting on Monday morning.

Flying from north to south or vice versa does not have the same effect on time changes and the circadian rhythms are not disturbed. However, in such cases there is likely to be a marked change in climate, and travelers should always give attention to the choice of appropriate clothing and to a marked increase in fluid intake.

OTHER FORMS OF TRAVEL

What about the medical hazards of other forms of travel? The common frustrating—and therefore extremely tiring—factor in travel both by train and by car is overcrowding and congestion. Many executives make a point of missing city rush hours by arriving early and leaving late, and flextime, flexible working hours, has made a big difference to less senior members of many staffs. They are able to work so that at least they might miss the rush hour one way. Anyone whose work entails regular driving over fairly long distances, perhaps covering many thousands of miles a year, should stop at regular intervals on each journey. The same rules apply as in flying, although to a lesser extent—having small regular meals and a good intake of nonalcoholic drinks.

IMMUNIZATION FOR TRAVEL ABROAD

It is always wise to check the regulations for vaccinations and inoculations for entrance to various countries, as these do change from time to time. This information can be obtained from the U.S. Passport Office. It is better for the traveler to space the vaccinations out and to recover from any minor side effects well before departure, and it is therefore sensible to make inquiries a month or two ahead if possible. Secure Americans tend to forget that in much of the world infectious diseases are still the main public health problem. Outside Europe travelers will be exposed to poliomyelitis and diphtheria as well as the more exotic tropical diseases. Whatever the age, anyone going further afield than Europe and North America should make sure that he has been immunized against polio (two or three doses of vaccine taken by mouth), diphtheria, and tetanus.

TROPICAL DISEASES

The World Health Organization, after an enormous campaign over many years, has eradicated endemic smallpox except for a few isolated areas in Ethiopia. This is a great achievement; however, many countries still insist on a vaccination certificate, which must be renewed every three years. With a revaccination, the certificate comes into effect immediately; a primary vaccination (one performed for the first time), is not effective for eight days. An international vaccination certificate has a doctor's signature validated by the local health authority community physician. Lack of a valid certificate can still interfere with travel in certain countries.

Cholera
Cholera is a disease of defective hygiene that in recent years has spread to the Middle East; almost every summer there

are also a few cases among vacationers returning from Mediterranean areas. Vaccination, which gives useful protection, requires one injection every six months. Again there is a special international certificate, which may be necessary for travel to certain countries in which there is a current outbreak of the disease.

Yellow Fever

Yellow fever is found in parts of Central America and Africa. The vaccine is a live virus, and the inoculation must not be given at the same time as smallpox vaccination—there should be an interval of at least three weeks between the two. Yellow fever vaccination can usually only be obtained from your doctor. Again an international certificate is available; it lasts for ten years.

Hepatitis

Virus jaundice or hepatitis is one of two or three serious health hazards for the American traveler to an undeveloped country. It is especially common in India and further east. The disease is spread by food and drink contaminated by defective sanitation, so the risk is greatest for the traveler who moves away from international hotels and restaurants. Vaccination, which gives partial protection against the disease, is available; a single injection is effective for about six months.

Typhoid

No countries require typhoid and paratyphoid A and B vaccinations, but they are a wise precaution for a family going to live and work for any length of time in countries in the Far East, India, Pakistan, and the Middle East.

Malaria

Vaccination is not yet available against the most dangerous disease for the international traveler, malaria. Each year several thousand people fall ill on their return from trips to Africa and Asia and each year there are tragic deaths—tragic because malaria is a preventable disease.

Malaria is still prevalent in most countries in Africa, Asia, the Far East, and Central and South America. The disease is caused by parasites which multiply in the bloodstream, and infection is transmitted by mosquitoes. A single bite by an insect carrying the disease is enough to pass on the infection, and there is no way that even international-quality hotels can keep out all mosquitoes. The disease is dangerous because there may be no symptoms for days and even weeks after exposure, and once back at home the businessperson may not connect sudden illness with a trip abroad the previous month. About one quarter of the cases reported by Americans are of the malignant tertian form of the disease, by far the most dangerous type. Malignant malaria can block the blood supply to vital organs including the kidneys and the brain, causing brain damage or death within a few hours of the onset of symptoms.

Protection against malaria is, however, simple. All that the traveler needs to do is to take a dose of a suitable anti-malarial drug once a week starting one week before leaving home, during the trip, and for a *full month after returning.*

TRAVELERS' DIARRHEA

By far the most common complaint among tourists and business travelers is diarrhea. Its frequency is obvious from the range of names for the illness: Aden gut, Basra belly, Delhi belly, Montezuma's revenge, and the Aztec twostep; and the distinguishing feature of this form of diarrhea is that it affects newcomers but not residents. Research on groups of athletes attending the Olympic Games and on servicemen has shown that the diarrhea is due to a minor infection with bacteria to which local inhabitants have become immune. In theory travelers should not become infected if they eat only in hotels and restaurants with high standards of hygiene, but few people completely escape infection during a stay of three to four weeks in an unfamiliar country. On a short stay of a day or two it is worth not eating foods that have a high risk of contamination. Fruits and salads should be avoided, and cold meats are also a potential hazard; it is best to choose freshly cooked foods. The water should be boiled for safety and kept in a refrigerator, and in a restaurant it is better to drink bottled mineral waters of a known make, and to avoid ice in drinks.

The chances of an attack of travelers' diarrhea may be reduced by precautionary treatment with an antibacterial drug available on a doctor's prescription. Clearly such treatment is not usually reasonable for a stay of more than a few days, but someone flying to, say, Cairo for a week may wish to make sure that he does not have diarrhea for the most important forty-eight hours of his stay.

OTHER INFECTIONS

The infection acquired most often by travelers is, however, not one of the tropical diseases or an intestinal disturbance; it is one of the venereal diseases. Worldwide, gonorrhea is now the most prevalent bacterial infection, and in many countries the risk of infection is very high. The precautions are obvious.

SUNBURN AND ACCLIMATIZATION

Sunburn may seem a trivial problem, but it is a recurrent one, and while a traveler may become experienced his skin has no memory. After a few months of a northern winter the skin takes forty-eight hours to acquire any protective tan, and for the first two to three days in strong sunlight protection is needed against direct exposure.

Just as the skin takes time to adjust to a change in climate, so does the body. The internal thermostat has to reset itself to cope with a higher air temperature, and it takes a few days for sweating, production of urine by the kidneys, and other biological mechanisms to become modified to the new conditions. During this time any heavy exertion—playing tennis, climbing a hill, playing eighteen holes of golf—will prove very fatiguing, and indeed there is a possibility of heatstroke. As with the change in body rhythms, the only solution is patience; the internal mechanisms will adjust, but they take time to do so. Again, the process will be eased by attention to fluid balance—plenty of soft drinks, not too much alcohol—and plenty of sleep.

MEDICAL AND INSURANCE COVERAGE

For those traveling on business, insurance against medical expenses will in most cases be arranged by the company, but if one or more of the family is on the trip a private arrangement may need to be made. Most people have no idea how expensive it is to be ill away from their own country and medical insurance benefits.

ON RETURN

Travelers should not expect to arrive back at home on, say, a Sunday evening and bounce back into the office Monday morning. Traveling is always tiring, and its effects are made worse by changes in time zones and climate. It is important to allow as much time to readjust on returning to America as was needed to settle into the country visited.

Finally, should any symptoms of illness develop in the weeks after a foreign visit, the doctor should always be given details of the trip abroad. There are many minor tropical infections, easily treated with modern drugs, which would not normally be suspected and would not even be considered as the cause of the illness unless the doctor was aware that the patient had been abroad.

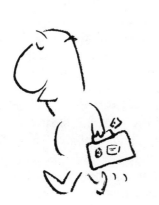

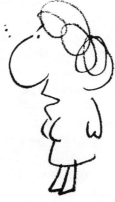

Remember that other women may count as leisure — but they aren't good for you...

chapter 10
LEISURE: A LUXURY YOU MUST AFFORD

WHAT IS LEISURE?

The casual reader of the Sunday newspapers' color supplements may be excused for having come to the conclusion first, that leisure is something to do with the pleasure of drinking rum on a tropical beach, and second, that there is little leisure in his life. In fact, the word "leisure" is derived from a Latin stem which means things which are *permitted.* The early English use of the word meant an opportunity to do something, and gradually the use of the term has changed through a "state of having time at one's disposal" to "free time." When we think about leisure, it is useful to keep in mind the various meanings the word has had.

One thing that is immediately evident is that leisure is not synonymous with pleasure. One person's leisure activity is as often as not another person's work. Gardening, playing the violin, even clearing a blocked drain, may be relaxing occupations for an executive who has spent his week behind a desk, but not for a gardener, musician, or plumber.

Leisure for most people is a fairly new concept. There may once have been a "leisured class," but its members, like the idle rich, have now largely disappeared. Most of our grandfathers worked every Saturday, and probably most Sundays as well. Those Sundays that were free were occupied by the Church, and fifty years ago it would have seemed strange for a book about health to devote a chapter to the problems of leisure. Even today, filling excessive leisure time will probably not be a problem for many executives, as few can follow the pattern of the leisured class and pay someone else to tend the garden or cater entirely to the needs of children.

CREATIVE LEISURE

Household chores of this sort may provide the executive with distractions from work, but they are not necessarily the most profitable ways of spending leisure time from his own point of view. It does seem to be accepted that the pace of life has significantly increased in recent years, causing a new kind of strain on many of those whose work involves heavy responsibilities, tight deadlines, long hours, complex work, or decision-making. In order to combat the draining effects of this life, the executive should make time to pursue positive leisure activities. The habit of working over-long hours is a difficult one to break; it is often made early in the executive's career, when the need to prove himself or herself to superiors by achieving more than is perhaps expected is a strong drive. Most people in executive positions thrive on the stimulus of pressure, but beyond a certain point the pressure becomes a cause of anxiety, the long hours become a burden, and the level of fatigue rises. To avoid the onset of any of the attendant problems already discussed in previous chapters, the answer may be to find more time for enjoyment. A tired executive does not necessarily require only sleep; a change of scene may be needed— he or she may need leisure, both for personal well-being and for the sake of the company.

The hours worked by people in certain jobs—such as piloting airliners and driving trucks—are controlled by law, because it is well established that excessive hours at work lead to the reduction of efficiency and thus of safety. Doctors certainly make mistakes when they have been on duty too long, but their hours are not controlled. It has not yet been convincingly demonstrated that the overworked executive is a danger to the company, but it seems reasonable to suppose that he or she may be. If not actually dangerous, performance may become stale and below par.

To avoid fatigue we need rest, but to maintain peak efficiency we also need a change of external stimulus. One of the undoubted benefits of regular exercise is a general improvement not only in physical agility but also in mental well-being. This is difficult to quantify, but it may well be the most important reason for improving one's state of physical fitness. A change of stimulus can also be provided in other ways. Regular chess, embroidery, photography, music-making or concert-going, theaters, the movies, bee-keeping, gardening—any activity that provides an absorbing interest which is quite separate from work can lead to much the same state of mental well-being as can physical exertion. It is of course not possible to recommend suitable interests in the way that a program for achieving fitness can be described; nevertheless, the value of developing and maintaining such pursuits cannot be overemphasized.

There are people who find it difficult to stop thinking about their work, and who tend to feel guilty when they relax. They are likely to be more competitive than others, and are commonly found in the upper reaches of a company or profession. They may be more likely to push themselves to their limit, but there is not much hard evidence that those who find it difficult to relax are at any positive health disadvantage compared with their more easygoing colleagues. Nevertheless, common sense would seem to dictate that a totally single-minded person may find it harder to absorb disappointments, to adjust if things go wrong. In addition, it does seem to be true that for many people paying attention to physical and mental well-being actually improves their working performance.

APPROACHING ACTIVE LEISURE

Although a certain amount is known about the relationship between activity and diseases such as heart attacks, and although quite a lot is known about activity and physical fitness, virtually nothing is known about the medical aspects of physical fitness, and it is important not to confuse the two.

Several studies have identified heavy physical activity as apparently protecting men from heart attacks. This finding has not been universal, but possibly differences have arisen because different activity levels have been compared. The best-known study was that of London busmen, which showed that bus drivers had more heart attacks than conductors: the drivers sit all day behind the wheel, while conductors rush up and down the bus, so obviously—the simple explanation goes—exercise is the important factor. However, this example also demonstrates the difficulties of this sort of study. At the time of selection for employment, drivers had to be issued with larger trousers than conductors, which suggests that fatter men decide to be drivers and thinner ones to be conductors. The risk of heart attacks is therefore possibly related to their original shape rather than to the activity of the job. There are other examples, though: in Finland, where heart attacks are common, lumberjacks seem to be relatively immune. In America, dockers engaged in really heavy work have been found to have a relatively low heart attack rate, although dockers involved in only moderate activity fared no better than sedentary workers.

As far as leisure time activity is concerned, a study of London civil servants has suggested that vigorous exercise on the weekend may be associated with a reduced risk of heart attack. The activities classified as vigorous included swimming, tennis, hill climbing, and the more active varieties of sailing; keep-fit exercises, heavy gardening such as clearing scrub, felling trees, and heavy digging; constructional activities like building stone walls and breaking up concrete; and climbing 500 stairs daily. Less vigorous activities such as cleaning the car, painting and decorating, cutting the lawn, and playing golf do not seem to be associated with a reduced risk of a heart attack.

One problem of the association between heavy exertion and a reduced risk of heart disease is that people who are physically active tend to be slimmer, to have a lower blood pressure, and to have lower blood cholesterol levels, all of which are themselves associated with a reduced risk of a heart attack. Some evidence suggests that the apparent effect of exercise is related to those other factors, while other evidence points to an independent role for exercise. Probably regular vigorous activity is associated with a reduced risk of heart attacks in its own right, but the association is less strong than is that between heart attacks and obesity, smoking, high blood pressure, and blood cholesterol level.

If we accept for the moment that vigorous, but not moderate, activity is associated with a lower risk of heart attacks then one obvious assumption is that the key difference between vigorous and moderate activity is physical fitness, for fitness only results from vigorous activity.

How Fit is Fit?

Physical fitness is a relative and not an absolute state: anyone from an elderly invalid to an athlete just short of Olympic perfection can be made more fit. Physical fitness is defined as a state in which more activity can be accomplished for a given amount of work by the heart. The heart rate is a crude index of heart work: fit people can undertake more exercise than unfit people without increasing their heart rates, and for a given increase in heart rate can do more exercise. In the attainment of physical fitness a law of diminishing returns operates: someone who for some weeks, perhaps because of illness, has undertaken essentially no activity at all can improve his state of fitness somewhat by very mild and simple exercise, but an athlete already in training must work very hard indeed for a minor improvement. For the average person to become significantly more fit a remarkable amount of exercise is required; exertion is needed which will cause mild breathlessness and sweating for thirty minutes three times a week.

The type of exercise is important. It must be "dynamic" and not "static," which means it must involve the movement of muscles and must not consist of straining against an immovable object like a stuck car or a heavy weight. Not only does static exertion fail to produce a state of physical fitness, it can also be positively harmful for it can be associated with quite dramatic rises in heart rate and blood pressure which may not be obvious at the time.

In one sense, physical fitness is like money—you have to work hard to get it. In another it is not—you cannot put it in the bank. Physical fitness is very rapidly lost and a deterioration can be detected after only three days in bed. There is no point at all in undertaking a program of training unless there is the will and opportunity to continue with at least three twenty-minute sessions every week. It does not require a very scientific study to show that for the vast majority of would-be sporting enthusiasts this is an unrealistic goal for more than a few months.

But for those with hope and determination to increase their state of fitness it is worth considering what sort of exercise should be undertaken. In simple terms, activities that do not induce sweating and breathlessness will not achieve much. Gentle walking and golf clearly rate rather low in the fitness league, while keep-fit classes, jogging, tennis, and squash are all more productive. The precise form of activity is unimportant provided it involves dynamic and not static muscle work; the individual can select the activity most suited to his inclinations, his available time, and his pocket.

It is, however, prudent to work up slowly through graded exercises, on each occasion not doing any more than induces the sweating and mild breathlessness that seems to be the best simple indicator of the right amount of work. Sudden extreme exercise is imprudent, and possibly particularly so in cold weather: shoveling snow has been reported to be associated with a high frequency of heart attacks, and the middle aged are perhaps well advised either to take an increase in their activity slowly and seriously, or to maintain and enjoy their accustomed sloth. Courses of supervised exercise for the middle aged are now becoming common, and form a good way of starting on the road to physical fitness. There are, however, some conditions in which exercise is definitely undesirable; anyone who has doubts about whether or not to embark on a fitness program should consult a doctor.

SEX: BETTER THAN A TONIC!

There are no medical conditions that make it unwise to have sexual intercourse. It is a fact that patients who have had heart attacks are frequently worried that sex may induce another attack, but there is little evidence that this is so. While in young, healthy people, intercourse can lead to quite dramatic rises in heart rate and blood pressure, these are not necessary and may well be less pronounced in the middle aged. The development of angina during intercourse is obviously an indication that the heart is being unduly stressed, but it is more sensible to seek medical treatment that will prevent angina than to avoid intercourse. There is not a fixed period of necessary abstinence after a heart attack. As soon as the patient feels like having intercourse the body is probably ready for it.

Similarly, there are not many medical conditions that make sexual intercourse impossible. Women may be inconvenienced by a variety of gynecological disorders, but all are amenable to treatment. Impotence in men can result from disorders of the nervous system, but the only common disease that causes impotence in middle-aged men is diabetes. Even in diabetes, impotence is often more a problem of general ill health than of specific nerve damage. Quite a lot of drugs (particularly some of those used for high blood pressure) can cause impotence, and anyone who thinks a drug he is taking may be having this side effect should consult his doctor.

The vast majority of men with impotence have no detectable organic disease and are not under medical treatment. Here the impotence is called "psychogenic" for it is presumably due to psychological causes. Fatigue is probably the main problem, and a period of real leisure is the best form of treatment. Patients troubled by impotence should not delay seeking advice for too long, for once it has been present for eighteen months or so the chances of improvement become steadily more remote.

EATING FOR PLEASURE

Now that malnutrition and vitamin deficiencies have almost disappeared from Western society, there are very few conditions of ill health in which the choice of food matters; there are many where the quantity consumed is of paramount importance. In the days when few real treatments were available for any disease, great store was set by the correct diet: it was believed that bland diets were good for ulcers in the stomach or duodenum, that rich foods were bad for gout, that eggs were bad for people with protein in their urine, and that salt was bad for everything.

We now know that no particular food is either good or bad for an ulcer, but rather that frequency of feeding is important; that diet is not necessarily related to gout; that there is no point at all in restricting the protein intake just because protein is appearing in the urine, and that while salt may be bad for people with heart failure (though not for those with any other common disease) it can easily be removed from the body with a drug that makes the kidneys excrete it.

Eating can be a pleasure in itself, and because it is often combined with enjoyable social occasions, celebrations, and so on, has an element in addition to the physical one of taking in food and appreciating the taste. The main problem associated with eating is that of obesity, which as readers will have discovered is one of the major causes of many aspects of ill health. There is, however, no reason why an interest in food should be denied because of this: develop an interest in the *quality* of food rather than in consuming it in large quantities, and the enjoyment is there without the dangers of overweight. This might even lead the executive to take up cooking—as an art, rather than as a chore. As a leisure activity the pursuit of better eating may provide the sort of change in stimulus that was discussed at the beginning of this chapter; the goal of which is to encourage the executive to lead a life sensibly balanced between work and leisure pursuits in a desire to maintain his health.

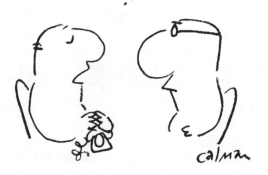

Do you consider yourself 'senior' or merely 'old'?

calman

chapter 11

THE OLDER EXECUTIVE

The nineteenth-century German playwright, Oscar Blumenthal, had his own view of the signs of being not so young. "A man," he explained, "is as old as his wife looks." The contemporary woman might reasonably add, "and vice versa." Certainly our first hints of the passage of time affecting us may come from observations of aging in those closest to us.

Fortunately for all of us, there are no absolute parallels between the number of years lived and the physical or psychological markers of time's effects. The current life expectancy for men and women lies between sixty-eight and seventy-four years, with the women doing rather better than the men.

In theory, then, the "middle age" period of life should lie between forty-four and sixty-four years old, but any boardroom observer will tell you that there are sixty-year-olds who look like fifty and forty-year-olds who look nearer sixty. The variations have multiple causes: inherited youthfulness or inherited premature aging, acquired weight excess or constitutional leanness, exercise or lack of it, weather exposure, occupational stresses, illness or good health, dynamic or static attitudes, and social role and social class. All these elements can influence the markers of passing time.

SIGNS OF AGE

There are several features of physical appearance that give useful clues. Greying of the hair on the scalp in both sexes is one feature, although some individuals go grey sooner than others, and a few will keep their hair color until they are elderly. In men, thinning and baldness are markers but here particularly the genetic element known as "male pattern baldness" confuses the aging factor. Hair thinning of this kind in women only occurs after the menopause.

Lines and Wrinkles

There are noticeable changes in the skin. Apart from any weathering effect related to much exposure to sunshine, there is a steady loss of elasticity. This is expressed in the wrinkles and folds which gather around and below the eyes, around the mouth, in the forehead, and in the region of the neck and forearms. Brown freckle-like marks appear on the backs of the hands. The familiar bloom of youth in the skin lessens, though in women this is more noticeable after the menopause, when there is a decline in the protective female sex hormones.

The Need for Glasses

A subjective marker which executives particularly notice is a change in the ability to read small print of memos, agendas, and company literature. In the forties, the elasticity of the lens in the eyes is reduced, which alters the ability to focus clearly—the reader holds the paper further away in order to reduce blurring. Known as *presbyopia,* the defect is corrected by suitable reading glasses, which allow the reader to hold literature at the normal distance from his eyes. Those who already wear glasses may need to change to bifocals. Presbyopia appears earlier in some individuals but affects virtually everybody by the age of sixty. Thanks to fashion in contemporary glasses and contact lenses, the female or male executive need no longer forgo the pleasure of easy reading with correct lenses for the sake of vanity. In any case, continual squinting in order to attempt to focus is aging in itself, and makes for crow's-feet round the eyes.

A Change in the Voice

Another change may be noticed in those who spend a great deal of their lives speaking and addressing others, on the telephone or in dictation. The quality and timbre of the voice changes. This may take on a roughened, hoarser, or deeper tone, or—more noticeably in women—a thinner, higher pitch. This voice change is the result of thinning in the muscles of the larynx and loss of elastic tissue in the voice-box cartilages.

Middle-Age Spread

The muscles of the limbs and trunk may lose some tone, and typically the abdomen becomes more protuberant and paunchy in both sexes—the classic "middle-age spread." Springiness and firmness of step is less marked in some individuals, and there is some slowing down in mobility or pace. From the forties onward, wear and tear in the cartilages of major joints—knees and hips, for example—makes for some stiffness of the limbs after prolonged periods of sitting. This may also be noticed in the back of the neck because of the same arthritic process in the bones of the spine. A long spell at the desk or poring over reports may be followed by considerable neck stiffness and discomfort. Getting up and walking about the office, or consciously moving the head from side to side to look over each shoulder in turn once or twice during the morning and afternoon may relieve this minor nuisance altogether.

The Value of a Smile

Teeth changes, with decay and loss or obvious dentures, are very aging in both sexes. Executives who have paid regular visits to the dentist over the years and had good conservation work on their teeth know the real truth. Loss of teeth and the need for dentures is related to three factors: poor dental hygiene and care, an excessive proportion of sugar and refined carbohydrates in the diet, and lack of natural or artificial fluoridation in the drinking water. The first two factors are controllable by the individual. You may find that an electric toothbrush is a very efficient cleaner and saves time. A visit to the dentist should be made regularly every six months, whether or not trouble is suspected. General health can be affected, while poor cosmetic appearance, mouth odor, and undetected infection can all stem from bad or carious teeth.

Hearing

Changes in hearing ability, related to aging of the inner ear mechanism, rarely appear before the middle fifties except in some individuals with an inherited "early deafness" problem. The rate of hearing decline is otherwise variable. It is more noticeable for the higher range of tones, as measured in decibels, so that a woman's higher-pitched speech may be harder to follow than a man's lower-pitched speech. Multiple conversations and background noise aggravate this type of hearing loss. Expert advice should be sought if problems in hearing arise; an inconspicuous hearing aid may make all the difference.

Sudden Exercise

Another sign of aging is the change in the reserve capacity for vigorous and sustained exercise. This stems from two main sources. Breathing becomes less efficient due to loss of elastic tissue and from a lessened capacity for oxygen and carbon dioxide exchange in the lungs. Heart muscle activity can remain quite regular but some thinning may occur, with a reduced capacity for forceful and vigorous contractions. The less exercise is taken, the more difficult sudden exertion becomes.

The Menopause

In women, the most distinctive of the time markers lies in the arrival of the menopause. In physical terms, this refers to the cessation of the monthly periods because the ovaries shut down, commonly in the late forties and rarely later than the fifty-second year. The menopause can occur prematurely in some women. There is an associated fall in female sex hormone production which varies from one woman to another. The resulting physical effects are parallel with the degree of sex hormone decline. Loss of skin sheen may result, other external changes take place in the breasts, which may be reduced in size and firmness, and in the external genital and internal genital linings, which thin down and are less well lubricated. In some women, sweating and hot flashes are a problem.

Other upsets sometimes noted are headache, irritability, and insomnia, all of which may affect executive work and decision-making; more marked mental upsets can include anxiety, listlessness, and depression. There is no need for difficult symptoms to be ignored or struggled against: help should be sought from the doctor if it is needed.

Logically, if menopause changes are associated with a decline in the body's internal production of estrogen, then the answer to virtually all the problems should lie in hormone replacement therapy, often described as HRT. This brings us to a comparatively recent controversy in medical management. In the nineteenth century, the medical view was strictly one of not interfering with the decree of nature in womanhood. In the present century, the availability of synthetic sex hormones suggested that it was reasonable and safe to deal with the physical changes and symptoms of the menopause by treatment for a limited time with hormone replacement therapy. This short-term symptomatic relief involves taking, for example, one or two hormone tablets daily, for three weeks out of four. The subsequent "period" is a cyclical bleed: it is not due to a return of fertility. As the symptoms of the menopause improve over the months, the treatment may be gradually reduced and finally withdrawn.

The controversial alternative is for HRT to be given indefinitely to menopausal and post-menopausal women. Dr. R. A. Wilson, a champion of HRT, says that continuous estrogen therapy makes the menopause and its symptoms "unnecessary." He claims that it permits continuing sexual enjoyment, avoids skin aging, and reduces the changes in breasts and sexual organs. There are also less obvious protective effects against the thinning of older bones and the development of artery changes in the female heart.

However, the controversy arises because those gynecologists who are against prolonged and indefinite HRT advise that the hormones may be a factor in initiating, or even promoting, malignant change in the breast or in the womb. Their view has led other medical scientists to look for non-hormonal treatments for major menopausal symptoms. One group has tried a slow release tablet which contains combined drugs—ergotamine, phenobarbital, and the alkaloids of belladonna. This was found helpful in relieving sweating and hot flashes, headache, and emotional upsets. Similar help was achieved by another research team who used the drug clonidine in tablet form for the same symptoms. Neither of these tablets influences the natural physical changes already described.

A marked increase of body weight, particularly in the breast and waistline, is often blamed on the menopause. It is far more likely that the coincidental psychological changes or upsets promote excess food intake as a solace or "anxiety relieving" factor. (It is also easy to forget that alcohol contains a lot of calories.) If there is any accompanying depression, then a checkup is advised as the doctor may wish to add supportive tranquilizer or antidepressant drug therapy.

SEXUAL SENSE—AND NONSENSE

One of the myths among the received ideas on sexuality in previous generations was that in middle life sex rapidly declined. In fact, worldwide studies indicate that sexual activity in middle life can and does continue in quantity and quality. Even old age brings a much slower decline, with no fixed universal end point. The decline in estrogen hormone production in women at the menopause does not invariably indicate a shutdown of sexual feelings, needs, and the desire for outlet. In men, male sex hormone production (and the capacity for sperm production and fatherhood) continues into the seventies and even eighties and again there is no invariable cutoff in male sexual desires and need for outlet. In fact, psychological problems dominate sexuality and potency changes rather than sex hormone deficiency or organic complaints.

It is true that physical ill health can affect sexual feelings and potency in either partner. Bronchitis, arthritis, fevers, heart problems, and other illnesses producing major or minor disabilities can temporarily—or more permanently—lower sexual tension and needs. However, medical advice can help to limit unnecessary sexual abstinence, or advise on alternative methods of sexual activity—more relaxed positions, manual stimulus, mutual caresses, oral activities, for example. There is no scientific basis for the male superstition that too frequent ejaculation is "weakening." All that happens with frequent sexual intercourse is a temporary fall in the total number of sperm in each ejaculation. Neither is masturbation or nocturnal emission any less acceptable than coitus as sexual outlets for the unpartnered in middle and later life.

Potency Problems

Specialists in genito-urinary medicine or in abdominal surgery, as well as family doctors, are familiar with the fears of middle-aged men that sexual potency is falling away and that this problem may be accelerated by medical or surgical treatments for other conditions. For example, one problem that many men first experience in middle life is a disturbance of the prostate (a gland at the base of the bladder). This may be in the form either of a nonspecific infection or of so-called traumatic prostatitis, related to much sitting down on firm or nonyielding seating. This can in turn cause discomfort or aching and there may be associated burning when passing urine. The local discomfort and aching can interfere with the maintenance of erection and proper ejaculation.

Prostate enlargement in middle life may interfere with the urinary stream, making an operation for removal of the enlarged prostate necessary. The sufferer from an enlarged prostate, who is happily enjoying an active sexual life, may have heard that prostate surgery can result in postoperative impotence. Nowadays, with modern techniques, this is very unlikely, and if it does occur is usually the result of psychological upset. This in turn responds to psychotherapy, tranquilizers, and effective sex therapy counseling. There are some operations, and some illnesses, which do interfere with potency, but no one should accept aging alone as a cause for impotence.

Sex Can Be Better

The hormone changes associated with the menopause may alter sexual tension and the need for sexual outlet in some women. Sexuality may increase, with rising sexual responses. This is variously explained as being related to freedom from any risk of pregnancy; fears that the sexual partner may look elsewhere; a widening interest in her socio-sexual role as woman rather than as mother-cum-wife; new horizons and contacts opening to the post-menopausal woman.

Alternatively, a temporary or more persistent decline in sexual desire may be noticed. This is variously explained as being related to anxiety or depression at the loss of fertility and the symbolic departure of a youthful era; discomfort at intercourse from the changes in the genital linings; choosing the menopause as a useful "excuse" for giving up sexual activity that has never been of real interest; introspection over lost opportunities in terms of physically attracting alternative partners, becoming a mother, or being competitive in physical appearance in the feminine world.

For the male partner too, middle age is a time of sexual reflection and reassessment. He too may experience an upsurge in sexual tension, as he compares himself with younger men and feels a resurgence of former urges to compete. He may look for this by seeking sexual outlets with other (often younger) women.

Again, the years may have altered his socio-sexual attitudes to monogamy. Alteration in the partner's physical appearance, or disturbance through her menopause, may further augment his sexual drive away from his usual source of relations and outlet. Alternatively a decline in libido and reduction in sexual tension may reflect a variety of circumstances: a change of path in his own career and social circumstances with sublimation of sexual energy in new executive drive; using the opportunity of his partner's menopause to give up sexual activity which has been of minimal interest for a long period; changes in mental or physical health, for example a period of depression or an operation in the region of his genitalia.

Alterations in mutual sexuality can result in clashes between husband and wife, or in any regular sexual partnership. Certainly the risk of separation and actual breakup is greater in middle age than at any time since the early years of that marriage or partnership. A separation or divorce may, in that sense, be an age marker in the life style of the male or female executive. Fortunately, for those who wish it there are many sources of professional help for the shaky middle-age marriage. This is available not only from the traditional counseling of the marriage guidance organizations but also from a range of clinics and individuals offering therapy for sexual, socio-sexual, and marital problems based on contemporary techniques.

PREVENTION AND CONTROL OF AGING

The various changes of natural aging so far described may prove troublesome for the executive who experiences them in proportion to their degree and rapidity of onset. Preventive and prophylactic executive medicine is concerned with reducing both of these variables.

Longevity and its associated delay in natural changes of aging does appear to run down the generations of some fortunate families; there is evidence of an inherited or genetic element. However, not even the managing directors of top companies can choose their own parents, let alone their grandparents, so prophylaxis for executives in eugenic terms is out at present.

Cosmetic Techniques

Hair and skin changes can be retarded in a number of ways. The executive who feels that grey hair does not give an air of wisdom or distinction can join the many individuals who use hair colorant or hair dyeing to restore the original hue, or tint away some of the grey. Similarly, those who feel that thin or bald patches accentuate other aspects of not looking so young may wish to consider one of the three cosmetic approaches: a modern wig or toupee, a hair weaving process, or an actual hair transplant from the neck area to the scalp area carried out by a cosmetic surgeon. It may be that older people who retain a youthful appearance often have advantages in job acquisition, job competition, and job success.

Roughening and wrinkling of skin is accelerated by excessive exposure to sunlight, so sporting a good tan—by visits to sunnier climes or by exposure to ultraviolet rays—is a mixed blessing. The female executive may follow her sex's example in facial skin care with moisture-giving creams and lotions, and facials, though she should remember that too much make-up is more aging than too little. Modern make-up needs to be subtle. The male executive does not have this advantage: he is liable only to use soap and water, and after-shave. The decline in elasticity, with secondary wrinkling and sagging, can be countered by cosmetic face-lifts. Essentially this involves taking up facial slack and removing skin excess at the fringe.

We are not here making a blanket recommendation of hair transplants and facial cosmetic surgery as being either invariably worthwhile or invariably successful. Most of these procedures are very expensive. All involve the discomfort involved in any type of operation. Hair weaving, for example, may require quite frequent repetition. Anyone wishing to explore this field must make sure of getting advice from a reputable source.

Another point to bear in mind is that highly sensitive individuals are not going to be transformed by any cosmetic operations. The best cosmetic surgeons are as interested in why the individual is keen to have a hair transplant or a face-lift as in the likely physical success of the operation. In fact, some cosmetic surgeons may require or request a satisfactory psychological assessment before agreeing to operate. This can be important. One of the elements in the depressive illness of middle age may be an over-sensitive preoccupation with personal appearance which has not, before the mental upset, been of major interest. Cosmetic surgery in such circumstances might be operatively speaking most satisfactory, but would not correct or improve the underlying depressive illness.

For this reason, too, consultation with a family or company doctor before going for cosmetic procedures in any area may be worthwhile. The observant and interested physician can give continuing advice and treatment for disruptive psychological elements in the not-so-young which may remove the need for operative procedures. Some cosmetic techniques and surgery are not available on company medical benefits; but a referral to a reputable practitioner can always be made through the candidate's own doctor.

Taking a Deep Breath?

Changes in breathing capacity, if becoming marked, again call for a full medical check-up and probably an x-ray. Most breathing problems in executives are self-inflicted by cigarettes— yet another good reason for giving up smoking altogether. Regular exercise is helpful, too, and a physical education expert or physiotherapist can advise on suitable exercises to improve and maintain breathing function over the years.

Arthritic Aches and Pains

The increased likelihood of "rheumatic" complaints, that is, joint stiffness and diminished muscle tone, with greater liability to muscle tension, aches, and pain is for the obese a further incentive for weight reduction. Unfortunately the onset of arthritis may lead to a vicious circle of decreased activity—

gain in weight—loss of mobility—gain of more weight. A determined effort to slim may often have a dramatic effect on symptoms of joint disease. Warmth often relieves joint and muscle aches, pains and tension, and the value of hot showers, sauna baths, Turkish baths, and spa baths is much increased in middle life for this reason; but medical approval should first be given before relief of this kind is sought.

Again, regular exercise can be helpful, although the sufferer from wear-and-tear rheumatic complaints has to strike a compromise between overworking and underworking the joints. Now that severely arthritic hip joints can be replaced by man-made implants, many thousands of men and women have had their mobility restored, and anyone with progressive stiffness of one or more joints should have a specialist's assessment of suitability for surgery.

Hardening of the Arteries

One other important change that affects everyone, at a varying rate, is known as hardening of the arteries, or arteriosclerosis. The normally elastic and supple arteries become narrowed and more rigid, reducing blood, nutrition, and oxygen flow to tissues, cells, and organs. All the major blood vessels to limbs, heart, brain, and kidneys, for example, are affected but the progress of this change varies from one part of the body to another—and from one individual to another. Hardened arteries augment and accelerate all the changes of natural aging described earlier; the effect increases from the sixties onward but no one can forecast the speed of the increase.

On present evidence, there are several factors which can retard the progressive hardening of the arteries by arteriosclerosis. A high blood pressure accelerates the process and, conversely, lowering the pressure slows it—hence the importance of regular checkups, including blood pressure measurement. There are now extremely effective drugs to control high blood pressure. Similarly, an annual checkup can pick up the presence of undetected diabetes. Uncontrolled diabetes can also make arterial narrowing worse. Overweight due to overeating is another factor, while there is additional evidence that a diet high in animal fats may make the risk of atheroma—degeneration in the inner artery lining—more marked. Some doctors advise that vegetable (polyunsaturated) fats are preferable to animal fats, whether used in cooking, frying, or at the table. The last—and familiar—agent that damages artery walls is tobacco smoke.

THE ADVANTAGES OF MIDDLE AGE

If the picture of middle age so far has seemed one of gloom and decline this is far from the truth. There are many positive advantages to be savored and enjoyed. The executive in his or her middle years is still in the mainstream of commercial and industrial life, able to feel the pulse of daily working activities, and in close touch with the products and profits of his enterprise. He or she has achieved some, even many, personal ambitions, but still has goals and prospects to strive for.

If he or she previously took a radical view of working and social patterns, it is still possible to do so without merely being the rebellious individual for rebellion's own sake. He or she is no longer interested in reflecting contemporary or youth-oriented cultural views and attitudes, as if young people's needs, wants, and activities were the sole arbiters of success and progress. Now he or she can decide what elements achieve a personal satisfaction and fuller enjoyment, instead of feeling it is necessary to follow the popular trend.

The executive is at the top or near the top of his or her particular tree. In relation to seniority, he or she can assume a wide range of options, rights, and privileges. These may be economic, functional, or social perks of the job as well as prerogatives in policy, timing, decision-making, choice, and direction. He or she can influence people, affect the lives of many, and promote the lives of a choice or chosen few. He or she can teach some and still draw from others, guide some and follow others from a front position.

Indeed the successful executive is a fine example of what the physiologist Hans Selye first described as the "general adaptation syndrome." Professor Selye was talking about the remarkable body link between the powerful hormone controller, the brain's pituitary gland, the crisis-controlling adrenal glands, and the sensitive mechanism known as the hypothalamus. These are linked in a chemical and nervous mechanism which helps us to respond and adapt to stress and hazards and external problems. At its most acute, it activates muscle tone, steels the eye, readies the limbs, keeps the heart ticking fast, and controls bowel and bladder. The top executive has the most efficient and personally responsive of such mechanisms. He or she does not normally require any artificial bolster against stress used by lesser mortals, in the shape of excessive alcohol intake or excessive medication.

Competence and Productivity

Acquired skill and professionalism is well maintained in middle age. The expertise and cumulated specific abilities permit greater competence in crises and urgent decision-making. They also help the individual to tackle new situations and altered patterns in a potentially successful manner. There is a greater sensitivity to received information and ideas, and less interest in whether such information and ideas will reflect well on the executive in a personal sense than in their likely contribution to the enterprise.

While the time of maximum creativeness, originality, and singular thought is often apparent in intelligent people in their twenties and thirties, the middle years may well prove to be the most productive in the broadest sense. This is expressed in a variety of ways—as the leader of a team or as an entrepreneur; in the formation of policy or as a communicator; in finance or marketing, development, or production. What is more important, as our earlier look at aging changes and health particularly showed, is that those who retain good health show a greater productivity than those with even minor illnesses.

Material Rewards

The economic advantages of the middle years for the executive vary somewhat from one country to another. Taken overall, however, the balance between income and expenditure tends to be more favorable than in earlier years. Any mortgage on the home may have ended or be nearing its end. Expenditure on children has ceased or is certainly much reduced. The shrewd executive will have substantial assets of both the material and cash variety, as well as enjoying the monetary perks of a high position. Admittedly, world-wide inflation and various levels of high taxation in many countries may lessen the benefits of a high income. Even so, it is possible to enjoy a comfortable and expansive lifestyle that contrasts favorably with earlier years of drive or struggle. In the best sense, the successful executive in middle years can indulge leisure interests and favorite entertainments in keeping with an upper salary range lifestyle.

Greater Understanding

Among the rewards and excitement of the middle years lies this self-perception: that the learning processes and varied experiences have given the individual a greater insight and a better grasp of the realities of life. What is read, what is heard, what is argued, what is seen, and what is encountered—all are appreciated and understood in greater depth than in earlier years. Insight replaces surmise, sagacity replaces guesswork, foresight replaces hopelessness, and judgment replaces juggling with pros and cons. The middle-lifer knows well that he or she has a whole host of strategies to deal with problems, crises, and contingencies at home and at work. Personal guidelines have developed and matured and the days of trial and error approaches have gone.

Another feature of interest in middle years is the element of bridging that may be felt. Both at home and at work, the executive is better able to view the aspirations and puzzlements, the ambitions and preoccupations of younger people, set against the fixed views and acceptance, the lack of interest in goals, and the more limited interests of those nearing or at retirement. By looking back and looking forward, he or she can draw the best elements from junior and senior age groups. In that sense, middle life can be a working model for the heirs apparent and heirs presumptive in an organization or in an enterprise. At the same time, the executive in middle life has a greater affinity with the older man or woman who has been through this particular mill, has survived and reached the time of disengagement, and is moving out from the mainstream of working life.

The sense of freedom already noted may be even stronger for the female executive than for her male counterpart. Any limitations that the presence of children or the possibility of pregnancy may have placed on her career have now gone. She can apply more time and more energy than ever before, and can permit full indulgence of her talents. She can explore new paths, demonstrate resources and capacities that may previously have been untapped or held in check. Any competition that she chooses to join is no longer side-tracked by issues of physical femininity but instead she can judge and be judged fully on her executive merits. She can show just how well the mature executive handles the highly complex role and singularly sensitive position of the senior officer in a corporate structure, commander and controller of the business environment.

A SENSE OF PURPOSE

In this chapter, we have looked at the signs and features which indicate to oneself and to the observer that we are not so young. We have considered what elements are controllable, what influences can and do retard changes of aging, and which particular elements in our lifestyle can be altered or modified to make and keep us healthier in middle years. Finally, we have pondered on the many advantages to the individual executive that middle life brings with it. Arthur Koestler wrote: "Adolescence is a kind of emotional seasickness. Both are funny but only in retrospect." He was able to say this from the vantage point of middle years. I prefer the view of Sam Ullman, the Alabama civic leader, who looked back from the summit of four score years and ten and said: "Nobody grows old by merely living a number of years. People grow old only by deserting their ideals."

ADDRESSES

Adult Education Association of
the U.S.A.
810 18th Street N.W.
Washington, D.C., 20006

American Aging Association
University of Nebraska Medical
Center
42nd & Dewey Avenue
Omaha, NE, 68105

Dedicated to helping people live
better longer.

Alcoholics Anonymous
468 Park Avenue S.
New York, NY, 10016

American Association for the Study
of Headache
5252 North Western Drive
Chicago, IL, 60625

American Association of Retired
Persons
1909 K Street N.W.
Washington, DC, 20049

American Cancer Society
777 Third Avenue
New York, NY, 10017

American Dental Association
211 East Chicago Avenue
Chicago, IL, 60611

American Foundation for the Blind
15 West 16th Street
New York, NY, 10011

American Health Foundation
320 East 43rd Street
New York, NY, 10017

Devoted to promoting preventive
medicine.

American Diabetes Association
1 West 48th Street
New York, NY, 10020

American Heart Association
7320 Greenville Avenue
Dallas, TX, 75231

American Institute of Nutrition
9650 Rockville Pike
Bethesda, MD, 20014

American Medical Association
535 North Dearborn Street
Chicago, IL, 60610

American Mental Health Founda-
tion
Two East 86th Street
New York, NY, 10028

American Pain Society
Pain Study Group
New York University Medical
    Center
550 First Avenue
New York, NY, 10016

Promotes the control, management,
and understanding of pain.

Anorexia Nervosa Aid Society
101 Cedar Lane
Teaneck, NJ, 07666

Offers counseling and organizes
self-help groups.

Arthritis Foundation
American Rheumatism Association
3400 Peachtree Road N.E.
Atlanta, GA, 30326

Cancer Information Service
1825 Connecticut Avenue N.W.
Suite 218
Washington, DC, 20009

Family Service Association of
    America
44 East 23rd Street
New York, NY, 10010

Gamblers Anonymous
2705-¼ West Eighth Street
Los Angeles, CA, 90005

Institute of Hypertension Studies
7032 Farnsworth
Detroit, MI, 48211

Institute of Lifetime Learning
1909 K Street N.W.
Washington, DC, 20049

Mental Health Association
1800 North Kent Street
Rosslyn, VA, 22209

A citizens' voluntary organization
devoted to the fight against mental
illness.

National Association of the Deaf
814 Thayer Avenue
Silver Spring, MD, 20910

National Council on Family
    Relations   .
1219 University Avenue S.E.
Minneapolis, MN, 55414

National Council on the Aging
1828 L Street N.W.
Washington, DC, 20036

National Foundation for Ileitis and
    Colitis
295 Madison Avenue
New York, NY, 10017

National Heart, Lung and Blood
  Institute
National Institutes of Health
9600 Rockville Pike
Building 31, Room 5A52
Bethesda, MD, 20014

National Interagency Council on
  Smoking and Health
291 Broadway
New York, NY, 10007

Seeks to develop and implement
effective plans and programs against
smoking.

National Kidney Foundation
Two Park Avenue
New York, NY, 10016

National Migraine Foundation
5214 North Western Avenue
Chicago, IL, 60625

National Society for the Prevention
  of Blindness
79 Madison Avenue
New York, NY, 10016

Rotary International
1600 Ridge Avenue
Evanston, IL, 60201

Weight Watchers International Inc.
800 Community Drive
Manhasset, NY, 11030

INDEX

A

Accountability: and frustration, 38–39

Adaptation: and stress, 29. *See also* General adaptation syndrome

Adrenalin, 64, 69

Aging, 193ff.; advantages of, 206–10; control of, 202–6; and sexual intercourse, 199–202; signs of, 194–99

Aggression: and exhaustion, 64; and the workaholic, 82

Alcohol, 41, 49, 51, 61, 117; addiction, 128–30; availability, 135–37; consumption guide, 137; and drugs, 131; effects of, 130–31; and hangover, 119; and mood, 131–32

Alcoholics Anonymous, 134, 135

Alcoholism: personality and, 132–33; society and, 133–34; treatment for, 134–35

Amphetamines, 151–52

Anemia, 61, 76

Angina pectoris, 67, 74–75, 77

Anorexia nervosa, 103

Appetite: loss of, 103. *See also* Food

Arousal: definition of, 72; and exhaustion, 63, 76, 81; and hypertension, 97; reducing, 78, 79–80

Arterial disease, 61, 69–72, 205–6

Arthritis, 17–19; and age, 204–5

Aspirin, 12

Atheroma, 69–70, 71

B

Barbiturates, 148–49

Bates, H. E., 74

Behavior: effect on health, 59–60

Behavioral hazard, 4

Bereavement: and stress, 72

Blaiberg, Philip, 73–74

Blood pressure, 2, 59, 71; and exhaustion, 64, 67; high, 95–98; low, 95

Bowels, 121. *See also* Constipation; Diarrhea

Bronchitis, 76, 140–41

Brunton, T. Lauder, 96

C

Cancer, 160ff.; checks, 167–68; cure, 162–65; diet and, 168–69; lung, 70, 71, 140, 165–66

Cannabis (marijuana), 152

Cataract, 20–21

Checkup, regular, 3, 8–9, 167–68

Chest trouble. *See* Bronchitis; Tracheitis

Child: and working mother, 52

Cholera, 177–78

Cholesterol, 64, 67, 69, 70, 71

City Gym Research Unit of London, 90–91

Coffee: and hypertension, 71

Cold, 11–13

Colon, irritable, 124–25

Community participation, 83

Conflict, 5–6, 33–34; interhuman, 84

Constipation, 121–23

Contraceptive pill: and coronary breakdown, 71; and depression, 49

Convalescence, 79, 89–93. *See also* Rehabilitation

Coronary breakdown, 62, 67–68, 90, 141, 156; action against, 76–81; danger signs, 72–76; minimizing risk of, 81–89

Relaxation: techniques of, 89, 91.
  See also Leisure
Responsibility: and stress, 4–6
Retirement: planning for, 41–42
Rheumatism, 15–16; and the heart,
  61

S

Saliva, 104–5
Schedule, irregular. *See* Living
  rhythm
Self-knowledge: importance of, 87
Selye, Hans, 207
Sexual intercourse, 190; and aging,
  199–200, 201–2
Shop floor: executive relationships
  with, 34
Sinusitis, 11, 13
Sleep, 40–41, 149–50; importance
  of, 73, 78, 79, 88–89, 92
Smallpox, 177
Smoking, 3, 138–46; and abnormal
  tiredness, 75; addiction to, 141–
  43, 142; coronary risk, 70–71;
  and health, 140–41; and lung
  cancer, 70, 71, 165–66; social
  acceptability, 143; women and,
  51
*Social Role of the Executive Wife,
  The* (Helfrich), 43–44
Stomach upsets, 118–19
Stress, 7, 28, 70; and female
  executive, 51–57; and the gut,
  100–101; patterns of, 45–47;
  reasons for, 27–28, 32–45; and
  responsibility, 4–7; symptoms
  of, 7–8
Suicide, 2; and under-employment,
  35
Sunburn, 180–81
Swallowing: difficulty in, 109–10

T

Takeover: trauma of, 36
Taste, sense of, 106
Taylor, Lord, 70

Teeth, 103–4
Thyroid gland, 61
Thrombosis, venous, 67
Tiredness: abnormal, 73–74, 75
Tobacco. *See* Smoking
Tongue, 106–7
Tracheitis, 14–15
Tranquilizers, 150–51
Travel, 172ff.; air, 173–74; fatigue,
  6, 39–40; insurance, 181; tropi-
  cal diseases, 177–79
Triglyceride, 64, 67, 69, 70, 71
Tropical diseases, 177–79
Tuberculosis, 59
Typhoid, 178

U

Ulcer: duodenal, 100, 114–17;
  mouth, 108; peptic, 114–17;
  treatment, 115–17
Ullman, Sam, 210
Under-employment, 34–36
Uric acid, 64

V

Valium, 88
Varicose veins, 23
Ventricular failure, acute left, 67.
  See also Coronary breakdown
Vitamin, 13, 61

W

Weight-watching. *See* Obesity
Wife: supportive role, 43–44;
  working, 52–54
Wilson, Dr. R. A., 174
Woman: as executive, 45; and
  middle age, 209. (*see also*
  Menopause); single, 54–55;
  working wife, 52–54
Workaholic, 82
World Health Organization, 177
Worry. *See* Stress

Y

Yellow fever, 178